REFLEXOLOGY
HARMONY & HEALTH

welcome to a world
of wellbeing
through your feet

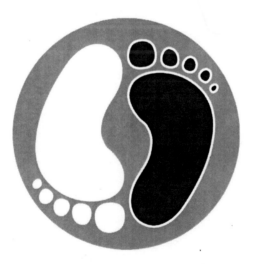

Sr. Brega Whelan

Sr. Brega Whelan

Reflexology: Harmony & Health

ISBN 978-0-9564602-1-9

1st printing , January 2010

Cover © Strega Design

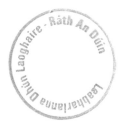

Published by
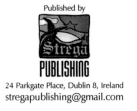
PUBLISHING
24 Parkgate Place, Dublin 8, Ireland
stregapublishing@gmail.com

REFLEXOLOGY
HARMONY & HEALTH

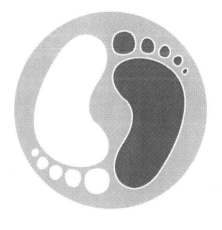

FIRST SECTION

SECOND SECTION

Reflexology and:

THIRD SECTION

FIFTH SECTION

FIRST SECTION

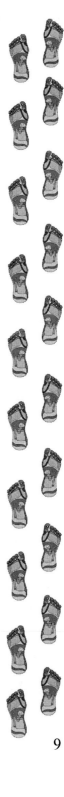

INTRODUCTION

For many years now I have been urged to write a book based on my experience of Reflexology in Ireland.

While taking care of the elderly patients in a nursing home, I met one lovely lady whose daughter, a nun with the Medical Missionaries, suggested to me initially that I do a course in Reflexology. I began training with one of their Sisters and subsequently attended one of the first courses in Ireland given by Jane Voudavik from London, who was extremely encouraging.

I had found my niche! I have continued to have a love affair with Reflexology since. I find this work so exciting and rewarding and the results so striking that while I have continued to do more courses, I now teach it to students from all over the world, in conjunction with my own work.

My hope is that this book will help to make this wonderful therapy better known and available to practitioners and non-practitioners alike, to students who will set up their own clinics, but also to the "man or woman in the street" ready and willing to help themselves and their families in the privacy of their own homes. I am a great believer in prevention and the way to achieve this is through Reflexology which restores the body's harmony and balance, thus allowing it to heal itself.

Unknowingly, we have all practised little bits of Reflexology, from a mother's stroking of a baby's feet to calm it, to the playful "This little piggy…" which works on the zones of the head in a fun way. The aim of this book is to show, in a simple way, the methods to help people to gain further insight into how they can help themselves to unlock the secrets of the feet, so that they are encouraged to take responsibility for their own health and thus be able to live a better, healthier, more relaxed life.

WHAT IS REFLEXOLOGY

Reflexology is a very natural, gentle, and safe form of treating the Body, Mind and Spirit in a holistic non-invasive way.

It does not aim to isolate any disease, but rather to try to get to the root of things, helping release disturbances and burdens in the body and re-establishing its own balance and harmony and allowing it to heal itself. Our feet have the ability to express our innermost feelings and sympathetically "tune in" to our thoughts and respond accordingly.

It works on the principle that there are specific points on the foot that correspond to the systems and organs of the body and by applying pressure to these points it is possible to pinpoint areas that are not functioning well, or have been affected by previous or present illnesses, or are blocked. Working these areas has been found to release the blockages in the energy flow, promoting changes which help to rejuvenate the body by restoring the normal balance. A naturally healthy body has beautifully formed feet, free of callous and blemishes. Distortions of the feet outwardly display distortions and misconceptions of the mind.

The marks of life's experiences impress both the soul and the sole and they are reflected on the feet long before being mirrored in the physical body.

A BRIEF HISTORY OF REFLEXOLOGY

Since ancient times Reflexology has been regarded as a therapeutic preventative practice. It is thought to have originated in China but there is visible evidence that it was practised in Egypt 5000 years ago, in the time of the pharaohs, since depictions of both hand and foot reflexology have been found in the tomb of a physician of that time. The native Indians of America also used it extensively to help heal their people. A form of Reflexology was known in Europe as far back as the 14th century with books published in Germany and Italy. Neurological studies were carried out in London and in Russia, where reflexes were being investigated by Dr. Pavel and others. But the credit for re-introducing Reflexology in the 21st century must go to an american E.N.T. specialist, Dr. William Fitzgerald, who found that pressure on specific areas of the foot had an effect on a related area of the body. He divided the body into 10 equal vertical zones, 5 on either side of a central line, stretching from the top of the head to the tips of the toes and fingers. He found that there was a direct link between a specific zone in the foot or hand which related to structures and organs of the body within that zone.

A pupil of his, Dr. Shelby Riley, refined these theories and added transverse lines to the longitudinal ones and wrote a book on zone therapy. But it was one of his assistants, Eunice Ingham, a nurse and physiotherapist, who charted the feet on her book "Stories the feet can tell" in 1938 and whose map of reflex points on the feet is still the basis of the therapy today. She is regarded as the founder of modern Reflexology and it was a pupil of hers who introduced it into Britain in the 1960s. Her nephew, Dwight Byers, promotes her methods holding seminars all over the world, as well as writing books on the subject and I had the pleasure of meeting with him after a talk he gave in Ireland many years ago.

We owe huge thanks to all of the people mentioned and many more, for passing on their knowledge of this beautiful, gentle therapy and for the contentment it has brought to people all over the world.

THE BENEFITS OF REFLEXOLOGY

Nowadays people are becoming more and more health conscious. There is a swing away from conventional medicine, which many perceive to have failed them, resulting in an increased demand for safer, more natural therapies, which are free of drugs.

For the body to be healthy everything must work together in a holistic, rather than a divisive way. It is becoming more apparent in this high-tech, supercharged world that preventative medicine is extremely important. Complimentary therapies based on this principle are widely practised, but they are never in opposition to conventional medicine, in fact they can work very well alongside each other. My personal belief is that Reflexology tunes the body up, so that it is better able to ward off stress, the major cause of illness. In fact psychological research has shown that any intervention that make a person feel less stressed, more valued, less rushed or even more confident, will enhance their ability to overcome symptoms of illness. Stress reduction has proved positive in making post-operative wounds heal faster.

Obstruction in the energy lines: Reflexology teaches that every organ and every gland depends for its survival upon its ability to contract and relax. When an obstacle is placed in the energy channels, as when acid crystals, waste, or unusual calcium deposits form on the delicate nerve endings of the feet, the energy flows is impeded and the organ it serves is then adversely affected. Obstruction in the energy line and fields register as pain in certain conditions and create limitations in motion and functions, for example a stiff neck or a painful back.

Energy blockage also interferes with blood circulation and this is usually first noticed in the extremities. Hands may become stiff, cold and often painful. Waste products accumulate at the lowest part of the body (because of gravity), which can be distinctly felt under the thumb and fingers as you work on the feet.

Reflexology brings peace and relaxation to the whole body, calms the mind and restores mental alertness, resulting in an overall feeling of well-being. There are no boundaries or limitations to its benefits. It is safe for everyone from babies to adults to the middle aged and the elderly of both genders.

A person doesn't need to be sick in order to benefit from Reflexology. People who have regular treatments have been shown to be able to cope better in general, are more placid within themselves, are less susceptible to minor ailments, have better circulation. Reflexology also helps to detoxify, to recover quicker from illnesses and from surgery; it benefits on many levels, not only physical and mental, but also the spiritual.

THE TREATMENT

The full treatment takes 40-60 minutes approximately, which includes relaxation procedures at the beginning and the end. There is a shorter version called: Vertical Reflex Therapy (V.R.T.), a variation on conventional Reflexology. It is a form of standing Reflexology (as opposed to sitting or lying down), which was developed by a British reflexologist, Lynne Booth, who discovered that weight or pressure on the feet gave better results. It is a very short, versatile and extremely effective treatment were the foot is worked dorsally (on the top) for a maximum of 5 minutes. It can be used on its own, or with a shortened conventional Reflexology treatment, which will take 20 minutes. It is used extensively in Britain in large department stores, with football teams, etc.

Each practitioner will know what is best for their client, based on the findings during treatment and will arrange follow-up treatment accordingly. However, having concluded a course of treatments, many clients return to visit their reflexologist whenever they feel they need help, simply to relax and de-stress from the normal day to day pressure of life.

REACTIONS TO REFLEXOLOGY

The main reactions immediately after treatment will be mostly pleasant, either calm or relaxed or energised and enervated. Because Reflexology activates the body's own healing powers to get rid of the toxins, some form of reaction is inevitable, but they are mainly cleansing of the elimination system.

As people differ, so will their reactions:

- There may be increased urination which may be darker and stronger smelling.
- There may be more frequent bowel movements and flatulence.
- There may be improved skin tone and texture, due to the improved circulation.
- The secretions of the mucus membranes of the nose, mouth and bronchi may be increased.
- Skin conditions may be temporarily aggravated with increased perspiration and pimples, or they may get very pale temporarily.
- Dependant on the depth of relaxation achieved, the client may feel like going to sleep.
- Sleep patterns may be altered and can be either deeper or more disturbed.
- There may be dizziness or nausea, which is temporary.
- Discharges from the vagina in women may be increased.
- Clients may feel tired, weepy or distressed, either immediately after the treatment or later.
- Others may laugh and feel very well, pampered, calm or rejuvenated.
- Previous viral infections may flare up again, in effort to heal.
- Physical reactions e.g. jerkiness of the arms and legs.
- Some people feel completed enervated and focused.

No therapist can predict or make any guarantees on what will happen after a reflexology section because this depends on each individual.

All people differ, so do their reactions: most people feel energized or relaxed, but some people might feel very emotional and cry. While old patterns can be released at a level that people can cope with, there can be significant changes in physical, mental and emotional health. Throughout the course of treatments, client may experience a sense of purpose in life. Reflexology practitioners are not just trained to treat, but also to listen to the words and what lies behind those words.

REFLEXOLOGY PRACTICE

Before treatment the Therapist will:
- Assure the person of complete confidentiality.
- Explain simply what Reflexology is.
- Describe and demonstrate the techniques to be used, sharing all information with them, being open, helpful and honest.

Explain that the Therapist:
- Does not diagnose or practise medicine and is not in competition with conventional medical practice.
- Does not advise, prescribe or adjust medication.
- Does not treat for specific illnesses.
- Does not heal, rather it is the body which heals itself.
- Suggest they see a chiropodist if they have foot problems e.g. verrucae, in-grown toenails etc.
- Alert them to possible reactions during treatment e.g. changes in temperature with sweating of the hands, feet or body, discomfort, sharp needle like sensations, which are temporary.
- Encourage them to self-help, which will help them to get involved and speed up results.

- Explain the possible reactions they may have.
- A medical check up may be suggested, dependant on what has been noted.
- After treatment a glass of water should be taken in order to flush out the released toxins.

REFLEXOLOGY ZONES

Reflexology derives from Zone Therapy. Dr. William Fitzgerald, who worked on the theory, found that the body could be divided into 10 longitudinal zones, five on each side of a middle line. These zones didn't cross the body, so the toe on the right side related to the right side of the brain, etc. These zones are not lines like acupuncture meridians, but are sections of equal width, through the body, extending from front to back. So whatever zone an organ is in, there is a corresponding reflex to that zone in the same zone of the foot. All of these zones are mirrored in both the feet and the hands, which contain reflex points that correspond to every organ, gland and part of the body. As well as the original 10 longitudinal zones, there are 3 transversal zones in the body and thus in the feet:

1) A line drawn across the upper shoulder girdle:
   at the base of the phalanges (for head and neck)
2) A line drawn across the waist level:
   at the base of the metatarsal bones (toracic area)
3) A line drawn at the pelvic floor:
   across the tarsal bone up to the ankle bone (abdomen/pelvis)

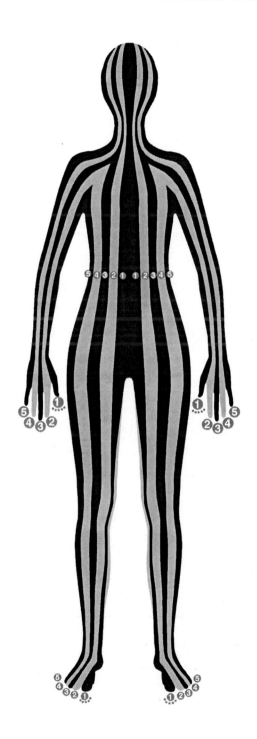

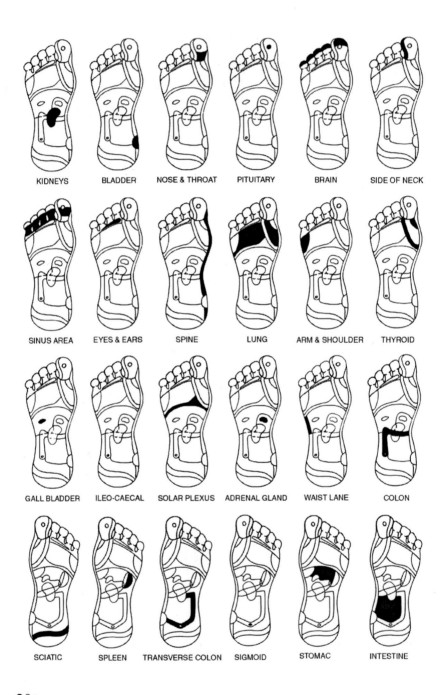

KIDNEYS   BLADDER   NOSE & THROAT   PITUITARY   BRAIN   SIDE OF NECK

SINUS AREA   EYES & EARS   SPINE   LUNG   ARM & SHOULDER   THYROID

GALL BLADDER   ILEO-CAECAL   SOLAR PLEXUS   ADRENAL GLAND   WAIST LANE   COLON

SCIATIC   SPLEEN   TRANSVERSE COLON   SIGMOID   STOMAC   INTESTINE

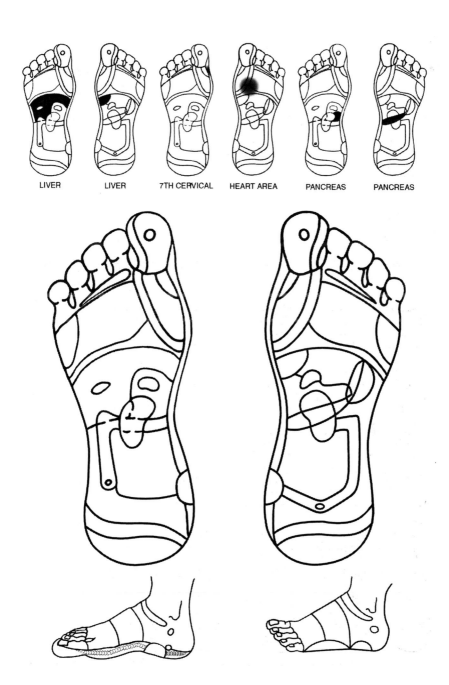

| LIVER | LIVER | 7TH CERVICAL | HEART AREA | PANCREAS | PANCREAS |

SECOND SECTION

Reflexology and:

1. Touch

2. Cancer

3. Terminally Ill

4. Stress

5. Infertility

6. Children

7. Elderly

8. Pregnancy

9. Animals

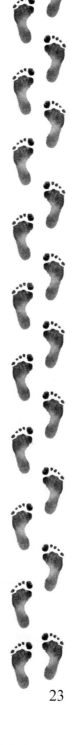

TOUCH

Touch, which is so vital to human beings, is taken completely for granted for a balanced well-ordered life. Until recently, this fact was completely ignored and misunderstood. It is now recognised that when touch is missing it can result in enormous difficulties.

We have many families with horrific pictures of children, abandoned at birth and brought up in institutions, whose mental and physical development was retarded beyond belief.

A move to a more caring environment ,where they were petted and hugged, brought swift and enormous changes for the better.

Is it well known and documented too, that premature babies in intensive care who are touched and caressed have a much greater survival rate than those who are not. Throughout nature all animals are very tender towards their young and this tenderness is most often expressed in touch. Both physically and psychologically, touch is an essential component that comforts and heals us, gives us a sense of security and helps with our development, our stress levels and ultimately our survival.

Reflexology and touch:

Touch is the most basic form of communication we know of and nowhere is this more evident that in the practice of Reflexology, where holding and touching the feet in a specific way has therapeutic effects which are legion. Reflexology differs from massage in that it accesses reflex points in the various zones in the feet, with an energy exchange between the therapist and the client. Kirlian Photographs has demonstrated that both the energy of the client and the therapist is increased during and after treatment.

Subconsciously, messages are conveyed through touch and any Reflexologist of experience will know, intuitively, which are the areas of the foot that are in need of treatment, in response to the pressure they receive through their hands. Many clients fall asleep having a great sense of security and total relaxation, engendered by the continuous contact and touching of the feet. They feel comfortable, at ease, relaxed and cared for.

Reflexology is a soothing way of touching, which is highly appropriate and does not overstep any boundaries. Those who respond greatly to the healing and caring touch of the Reflexologist include: premature, separated or abandoned babies, hyperactive children, traumatised or injured adults, the mentally disabled and the terminally ill.

CANCER

There is no disease so hedged about by anxiety and fear as cancer. For many, even the word cancer is so terrifying that it is only referred to by pseudonyms, like "the big C".

Fear is the greatest crippler of human beings. It can grip people to such an extent that it almost paralyses them and they loose their peace of mind. The fear is usually followed by panic, shock, helplessness, isolation and lack of hope.

Nowadays cancer is becoming an increasingly common complaint, with one in three people developing it. It is no longer looked upon as a single disease, but rather is a very complicated mass of varying diseases, which have many causes, many different effects and respond differently to treatment. Cancer cells vary from normal cells in that they undergo changes: one rogue cell develops the ability to multiply rapidly and then invades the surrounding healthy tissue causing tumours, etc. There are three main orthodox treatments at the moment: surgery, chemotherapy and radiotherapy, but what can be really successful, if a person has a positive mind, is the determination to get read of stress, even though it may mean to change an unhappy life situation.

The causes of cancer are very complex and well established: tobacco and alcohol abuse, difficult life style, bad diet, pollution and the environment as well as hereditary.

There is much that can be done as preventative measures:

• It is never too late to give up smoking and avoid passive smoking.
• Have moderate consumption of alcohol, which is linked to liver, mouth and throat cancers.
• It is important to eat more fibre, fresh fruit and vegetables and to cut down on fat consumption, as one third of all cancers may be due to diet e.g. bowel and breast cancer.
• Threat the sun with the greatest of respect, always wearing a sun block outdoors. Skin cancer is the second most common form of cancer in these islands. Fair skinned, red and fair-hair people are the most at risk, as are farmers who work outside for long periods. Likewise sun beds should be treated with caution.
• Working with radioactive materials, hazardous chemicals,

asbestos etc. requires great vigilance and a strict adherence to safety precautions.

Much has been done to conquer this frightening disease. The modern technique of using genetic fingerprinting is opening up unlimited possibilities. Apart from the physical effects, the psychological impact is now being realised, with the need for a greater positive attitude. Quality of life issues are now more important than heretofore and treatments other than those of conventional medicine are being looked at and examined. Complimentary therapies have integrated into the complete treatment, with more openness than has been shown up to now by conventional medical practitioners.

Reflexology and Cancer:

Reflexology is a gentle, non invasive therapy. It is holistic, that is it treats the whole body rather than treating cancer alone:

- It is soothing and healing and can comfort both the patient and relatives, who may be in distress and shock at having to face their own mortality. The deep relaxation it induces brings about a state of calm, leading to peace of mind.
- It is a very safe form of touch, without breaching any boundaries, especially for those who may be uncomfortable with physical contact, conveying love and care to the patient more effectively than verbal communication.
- It can convey deep personal contact at a time of great pain and loneliness. Where a person has difficulty in expressing

emotions it can often trigger off relief, tears, etc.

- It enhances relationships, especially with family members.
- It increases a sense of well-being and wholeness, leading to improved self esteem and acceptance.
- It affects the person at all levels, mind, body, spirit, reducing stress of shock and restoring calm, which helps them to deal with their lives and treatment.
- It has been said that it can reduce blood pressure and improve blood and lymph circulation; the body, hands and feet feel warmer.
- It can relieve constipation and help with bladder function.
- Sleep improves greatly in quality.
- It can help to reduce headaches and relive pain.
- It can stimulate the immune system.
- It can reduce swelling not due to infection.
- It helps the nausea associated with chemotherapy treatment.
- If done the day before the treatment, reflexology makes the person feel less tired.
- It improves the quality of life and the energy levels of the person.
- It balances the body.

TERMINALLY ILL

There is an enormous amount of fear, anxiety, guilt and rejection associated with passing from this life and the modern tendency is to do everything possible to stave off ageing and dying. It is much easier for people to shy away from all thoughts of it than to face up to it, so when there is a diagnosis of an incurable disease, it traumatises to such an extent that the patient, relatives and friends often feel very helpless in dealing with it and very often, both the person and the family, react by withdrawing physically and mentally. They do this to protect themselves and to insulate themselves in some way from further hurt and also because generally speaking they don't know what else to do. But by withdrawing everyone becomes locked into very separated compartments of isolation and loneliness, out of which it can be extremely difficult to break. This situation can be helped greatly by a hospital or hospice's use of positive care, where is defined as the active, total care patients plus their families, by affirming positive living instead of the negative dying or death. Its whole purpose is to get across to the patient that they matter and that the quality of their lives is more important than the length of their days and that it can be improved. Often there is too much about and not enough talk with the patient. Positive care changes all that. This invaluable assistance to the patient, family and friends helps them all to deal with the pain, anxiety and loneliness and assists them to achieve the highest possible quality of life. Importantly, it helps to restore control of the patients own lives.

Reflexology and the terminally ill:

• It benefits because it treats the body holistically, on all levels: physical, emotional, psychological and spiritual.

• If offers a soothing, calming supportive therapy in a safe environment.

• It invites the patient to stay in touch with their bodies at a traumatic time and to benefit from a comforting, caring, safe, gentle touch. Touching lets them know they are not alone at what is a very lonely, isolating time for them; it affords comfort and support and allows them to feel cared for as a person.

- Sleep quality is improved, as are energy levels.
- Improves circulation, warming cold hands and feet.
- It can bring relief in the case of oedema.
- It helps with digestive problems and with constipation.
- It improves breathing or helps to relieve pain.
- It can help to reach the letting go process. Even people in a coma, who retain acute hearing until the end, benefit from an affectionate stroking of their feet. At a time when families feel they can't do anything, they can. Touch with empathy conveys not only physical warmth but also non verbal messages of love, care and support flow between them. The tender stroking and massage of feet takes away the feeling of helplessness and inadequacy.

Usually it is sufficient to treat the feet for 15-20 minutes using mainly relaxation techniques. Often the patient will lie back and drift into a peaceful relaxed sleep, their face will show when it is advisable to stop. Relatives, friends and non professionals should be encouraged to give this treatment to the seriously ill. It creates closeness and a bond too deep for words, which is of benefit to all.

STRESS

It is not possible to remove stress completely, but it is possible to learn how to manage it. First identify what's causing it, pin point the source, write it down. For example it could be related to home and family, work, self induced, environment related, etc. If you cannot do this by yourself, look for help through a sympathetic G.P. with time to listen, or to a counsellor or practitioner of complimentary therapies, who will help you work out what's best for you and then try to:

• Separate the major stresses from the minor and eliminate what can be eliminated.
• Learn to say "no", especially to things that you don't want to do. Speak your own truth.
• Don't attempt to be all things to all people, it never works.
• Try to be more flexible and more open to change, be more aware.
• Watch your health. Many people, especially men, look after their cars better than their bodies.
• Eat regular healthy meals and not on the run. Start with a good breakfast.
• Cut down on fatty foods, sugar and salt. Read all labels carefully.
• Cut down on processed and junk foods e.g. tinned foods, coke, chips and burgers.
• Cut down or cut out smoking and coffee. Body vitamins are depleted by these, by antibiotics and other pills.

- Have a moderate alcohol consumption.
- Every day eat five portions of fruit and vegetables.
- Take supplements on advice and if necessary have allergy tests.
- Exercise, either in the gym moderately or in the open air. Try and get a minimum of thirty minutes of fresh air every day by walking, swimming, cycling, tennis, etc.
- Use leisure time wisely. Have hobbies. Do therapeutic courses like metalwork, craft work, gardening, glass work, yoga, cooking, woodwork, painting, flower arranging, fishing, aroma therapy, etc.
- Take regular rest breaks or holidays. Short breaks taken often may be more beneficial.
- Make time for yourself, family and friends and for sport like football, rugby, G.A.A, golf, swimming, etc.
- Listen to gentle music and sit peacefully, in harmony with it for twenty minutes.
- Learn to meditate, do visualisation, deep breathing, etc.
- Whatever therapy suits you, go for it.
- Confide in someone you can trust, who will accept you as you are.
- Be content with what you have. Settle for less. Don't make comparisons.
- Even if you cannot control external events, you can certainly control your attitude to them. The only difference between positive and negative is a thought and you can control that.
- Structure the day in a diary and make off each completed task. Prioritise. Do the difficult and unpleasant things first.

- Lighten up. Laugh more. Watch comedies on film or TV.
- One thing at a time. One day at a time. Cultivate living in the now.
- Forget the guilt of the past. Don't think of the anxieties of tomorrow.

Our spiritual side needs feeding and nourishing too. There is a spiritual crisis all over the world. People hunger for a meaning and purpose to life. There is a need for a higher vision of good, which will transcend the selfishness of the world. Find a way to contribute to that good and not just materially. One of the main causes of many health problems today is stress, which is on the increase. It can be triggered off by innumerable factors: physical, mental, emotional or environmental. Of itself it is neither bad nor dangerous. A certain amount is not only necessary but desirable, in order to function well. Indeed there are some people who thrive on it and who wouldn't function half as well without it. Many of the most successful people are those who have learned to respond in a balanced way to high levels of stress. It is not practical to think it can be removed completely, nor would it be prudent. The secret is in controlling it to a level that can be dealt with, is learning how to relax. Stress is responsible now for over 70% of G.P. visits and it is one of the commonest causes of absenteeism. Job stress is a growing phenomenon. Years ago counsellors dealt mainly with the unemployed, today however they deal mainly with full time worker. Many employees complain of alienation, anonymity and of being unimportant and dispensable, they feel that they are treated with very little humanity and respect. This leads them to believe that the inanimate products are more important than the people producing them. So much pressure is brought to bear on them to produce results, they feel burnt out before they are even forty and can't cope.

Stress is not confined to men in the work place. More married women than ever nowadays have to put in a full day work outside the home. They plan for and transport small children to creches and schools beforehand and return home to be wife, mother, nurse, cook and cleaner. Home based women are not immune either, being cooped up in a house all day, seeing and speaking to no other adult leaves many of them utterly frustrated and depressed. It is small wonder then that many today feel so trapped that they resort to tranquillisers, alcohol and other drugs to keep going.

Stress is a new buzz word for an old problem. Adults of other times may have been as stressed, but they don't appear to have been and old people would say that they were not. They lived in a more leisurely time, in a less frenetic world and had a lot of help from their extended families, most of whom lived near them. They didn't have to cope with consumerism, materialism and all the other present day "isms". Nor did they have to deal with the many and varied aspects of the huge modern technological advances, which threaten to swamp them in a vastly changed, high speed, high tech world. Long ago they had less money, but more importantly they had low expectations. Whereas today vastly increased expectations, plus instant gratification, leading to increased demands, puts intolerable pressure on everybody. More money, more leisure time, better health care and all found more comfortable lifestyle would appear to lead to more cancer, more heart attacks, more depression and more suicides than could ever have been envisaged. When stress goes beyond the bounds of acceptable levels then it could be said that the person is in a 'distressed state' and alarm bells, whether physical, mental, emotional or psychological, go off all over the body, in a warning effort to get it back into well-being and wholeness. Symptoms of stress are not always immediately obvious, but may be divided into the physical and psychological, broadly speaking.

Physical:

- Neck and shoulder pain.
- Lower back pain.
- Headaches and migraine.
- Throat and chest constriction.
- High blood pressure.
- Disease like colitis, irritable bowel, fibromyalgia, M.E.
- Teeth grinding.
- Indigestion.
- Constipation.
- Diarrhoea.
- Allergies like asthma, eczema.
- Insomnia.
- Fatigue.
- Restlessness.
- Frequent colds or flu.

Psychological:

- Relationship difficulties.

- Anger and aggression.
- Increased impatience, irritability.
- Depression.
- Fear, anxiety.
- Feelings of isolation.
- Lack of concentration.
- Guilt.
- Low self esteem.
- Loneliness.
- Pessimism.
- Increase dependence on tranquillisers, alcohol, drugs.
- Lack of harmony with self and others.
- Crying fits.

Reflexology and stress:

Reflexology can help with stress by creating a state of total relaxation, leading to an enhancement of the natural healing powers of the body. As the body relaxes:

- The stress and tension levels are reduced.
- The mind is calmed and mental alertness restored.
- A lessening of tensions leads to a reduction of minor ailments, like headaches, migraine, cold and flu, etc. It also leads to better elimination functioning.
- Removes congestion in the energy pathways.
- It helps to normalise organ and gland functioning.
- It improves blood and lymph circulation, reduces blood pressure.

- It stimulates the body to eliminate toxins, which improves the overall physical tone dramatically.
- Sleep patterns are improved, with a knock-on improvement in work performance.

With a lessening of stress levels many people feel re-energised and, as a result, feel able to tackle their problems with renewed vigour, are able to re-organise their lifestyles, so as to prevent difficulties from assuming mountainous proportions, they regain the confidence in their own abilities and they can cope better. Peace, harmony and calm overflow into relationships, both at home and at work and a sense of general well-being is created.

INFERTILITY

Infertility is a very complex issue and has many causes:

- Medical disorders (blocked fallopian tubes, endometriosis).
- Low sperm count and impotence.
- Hormonal imbalance.
- Unnecessary stress, anxiety in relationships.
- The pressure of trying too hard to have a baby.
- Poor lifestyle or diet.
- An increase in sexually transmitted diseases.

A thorough check up with a gynaecologist is essential for any couple who suspect they may be infertile. Blood tests and ultrasound examination can ascertain if there is a physical cause, like blocked fallopian tubes or endometriosis in the female and semen analysis can identify male infertility. It is estimated that one third of infertility is female related and one third is male related, with the remaining third due to both partners or unknown causes e.g. genetic. Infertility is a widespread issue now and demand for treatment has increased to such a level that there are now five specialist clinics.

Reflexology and infertility:

It can stimulate both the hormonal systems and the reproductive organs, especially when used on peak ovulation times. The treatment is begun a few days before ovulation and continued every day until 2/3 days afterwards for at least 2/3 menstrual cycles. In the male, Reflexology treatment over a period of at least two to three months has been shown to increase sperm count.

One of the greatest benefits of Reflexology is the deep relaxation it induces. This deep relaxation alleviates stress and tension, releasing energy, which helps to stimulate the reproductive organs and to normalise glandular function. If a couple could learn to give Reflexology to each other, they would experience a greater warmth and closeness in the relationship, which would lead to more trust and the greater sense of security that a woman needs to be physically receptive. It is essential for both parties to relax. The more pressure they are under "to succeed", the less likely it is that conception will take place without outside help (e.g. I.V.F. treatment or assisted insemination).

A mutual Reflexology session could be enhanced by taking a slow leisurely bath beforehand. Giving the body every chance to relax will help it to respond. The emotional cost of infertility is high. People take pregnancy for granted and don't understand the longing for a child, consequently this very private topic is not discussed openly. A Reflexology treatment with a sympathetic therapist can provide the listening ear that may be required to help to overcome the feelings of isolation and sometimes despair.

CHILDREN

Reflexology benefits children in many ways. Holding and touching their feet is a special form of communication, which leads to closer bonding and gives a child a sense of security and of being loved and cared for. It is excellent for both physical ailments and psychological traumas of growing up. It is used to ease and get rid of accumulated stress whether it is:

• The stress of growth or growing pains.
• The stress of injury to young limbs.
• The stress of minor ailments or chronic conditions.
• The stress of life in general.

It is especially good for children who:

• Are not touched or hugged enough.
• Are abused either physically or emotionally.
• Are hyperactive, as it calms them.
• Are slow, as it can stimulate or energise them.
• Are handicapped, mentally or physically, as it helps their
   bodies to get back into balance and improves their behaviour,
   alertness and attention span.

It opens up avenues of communication between therapist and child, as very often during a session children will blurt out whatever is worrying them at school, or in the home, or with their friends. It has a preventative action in that it helps to boost their immune systems:

- Babies gain weight and sleep better.
- Bed wetting is controlled, constipation is reversed.
- There are fewer colds and throat and ear infections.
- Asthma and other allergies are controlled.
- Relationships with parents and friends are enhanced.

This is especially beneficial to teenagers, as puberty can be such a difficult time for them. It helps them to cope better with hormonal changes, with fatigue, with the stress of exams and athletics.

"Little and often" is a good maxim with children. They have a very short attention span and will only co-operate for a brief time, ten minutes maximum. The therapist can be much more flexible with the children than with adults and can treat them whenever or wherever it suits them. It is important to get them to accept the touch of hands on their feet from a very early age. In that way they are less likely to wiggle, squirm or jump away. They can be helped to co-operate by turning the treatment into a game or by enlisting their help in procuring a pillow, towel or powder.

Distractions can be kept to a minimum, but it may not always be possible to eliminate them completely, so they should be allowed to fidget and twist without annoyance on the adult's part. Punishment of any kind must not be contemplated. Rather, emphasis on gentleness, understanding and tolerance are essential for long term benefits. Self help too can be taught as they are very receptive, especially when they can see for them selves how effective this can be.

V.R.T. (Vertical Reflex Therapy) gives a totally effective treatment without tiring them, in five minutes.

Movement with babies should be gentle and unhurried. If a child becomes distressed, the therapist should stop and wait until the child is calm again. Although treatment touch needs to be gentle, too light a touch is irritating for most babies, but if the touch is too heavy, the baby will move their limbs away. When a session is over, the hands should be released lightly off the feet.

ELDERLY

Human life nowadays is rapidly becoming expendable and nowhere is this more apparent then in the treatment of the elderly. There is a culture of youth and everything young is acceptable, where anything old tends to be discarded. Society is strangely influenced by materialistic considerations and nowhere is there an acknowledgement of the foundations of our present affluence. The talent and energy of older people is undervalued. Their experience and expertise count for nothing as modern technology makes experience obsolete. Their hard won wisdom, which is an invaluable asset, is often overlooked or derided. While eastern cultures value their older people highly, the supposedly "advanced" western world believes that to be old is a burden and everything must be done to avoid it. Obsessed with their own youth and beauty, the young forget, or choose to ignore the fact that one day they too will have to accept the decline of their bodies and all that entails. How they behave now to their elders will one day be meted out to themselves by children, who by example have never been taught otherwise. Age is a time for reflection. It is a stage which can creep up on people and for which they have made no preparation. It is a natural process and it is part of the body's plan as it slows down. With age the immune system deteriorates, so the older person is more prone to illness, gets tired more easily and needs more rest.

There is little in the modern world that is admiring of age and advertisements and TV plug only youth and beauty. When they have to go to nursing homes the elderly find themselves uprooted, put into different surroundings among strangers, with young staff who may not understand them. It is very traumatic for them and they can easily become disorientated and troubled. When this happens then pills and tranquillisers are used to quieten them and to keep them trouble free.

Its far better for them if help is provided in their own home and environment, where they still have a measure of importance and can choose their own clothes, entertainment, music etc. to maintain their interest in themselves and in the world in general.

Despite the modern type of decrying age, there are advantages to advancing years:

- Views can be expressed freely without worrying about the opinion of others.
- Comfort is more important than fashion in dress.
- There is time, at last, to indulge themselves and start a course or pastime which always eluded them, e.g. theatre, art, travel...

- Each day is appreciated as it comes along and there is acknowledgement that every day over seventy is a bonus.
- The mind is concentrated by the single fact alone that the end of life is approaching and so doing is more important than procrastinating.
- The wisdom acquired throughout a lifetime is recognised, with a view to passing it on.
- The value of spirituality is noted and more appreciated, with the good outlook of longer and healthier lives.

PREGNANCY

The benefits of Reflexology in pregnancy are:

- It is a natural, non-invasive therapy which is painless.
- It induces calm and relieves stress.
- It is a means of bonding between mother and baby.
- It relaxes the baby in the womb.
- It reduces swelling of the ankles and feet (oedema).
- It helps with labour.

Reflexology is not recommended during the first trimester of pregnancy, but after that time it has been proven to be very successful and many midwives are now training to be reflexologist. The maternity hospitals find that, combined with the medical skills available, Reflexology is very valuable in pre-natal and ante-natal stages and it also supports and enhances labour.
Pregnancy is a time of major physical adjustment for the mother,

but also for the father who may undergo "a phantom pregnancy" in support and sympathy. Reflexology can be the means of releasing the attendant emotional stress in both, as well as benefiting the oedema, morning sickness and other attendance physical symptoms in the mother.

ANIMALS

Reflexology for animals works similarly as with humans, by using their "feet" and "hands". Some animals suffer the same stress related disorders as humans do, affected by noise, food additives and modern life. Animals have other similar problems to humans: weight, arthritis, diabetes, aches, pains and often stress.

When you work on an animal, remember that the paws contain reflexes to the head and chest. Working right up the leg, front sides and back, reaches reflexes to the bowel and stomach, liver, pancreas and spine.

THIRD SECTION

1. The Immune System

2. The Cardiovascular System

3. The Respiratory System

4. The Urinary System

5. The Digestive System

6. The Skeletal System

7. The Reproductive System

8. The Hormonal System

THE IMMUNE SYSTEM

The immune system is a collection of mechanisms, within an organism, that protects against infections and disease, by identifying and killing pathogens and tumour cells. It detects a wide variety of agents and needs to distinguish them from the organism's own healthy cells and tissues in order to function properly. The main components of the immune system are:

1) Lymphatic System
2) Spleen
3) Thymus
4) Tonsils

Lymphatic System

The Lymphatic System is crucial to the body as a method of waste disposal e.g. toxins and excess fluids. The system is a network of small transparent vessels, which parallel the veins and arteries, but it does not have a pump like the heart, so it cannot move on its own, it's dependent for its movement on the muscular system. Exercise, yoga, tai chi, walking, trampoline, dancing, sports, stretching or anything which moves the large muscles of the body will help the lymph's to move too. The system collects the fluid, which seeps through the blood vessel wall, filters it and returns it to the blood stream. Where vessels meet it has collection points or nodes, most of which are in the upper body, around the neck and under the armpits, though there are about one hundred of them all over the body. These glands swell in times of infection, as the body seeks to confine the infection to that local area and prevent it from spreading. Dead cells, harmful bacteria, viruses etc. are carried to these nodes, which then act as barriers to their further passage. The antibodies, which the body produces as a response to any invader, are made in the lymphatic tissue and are then released into the blood stream. The lymph can become stagnant as a result of no exercise e.g. in a long car or plane journey, when the feet and ankles swell. A stagnant lymphatic system can cause congestion in the nose and lungs, swollen glands, stiffness in the joints, over acidity, increased mucus and a lowered immune system. There are 2 main drainage points in the body for lymph:

1. The thoracic duct, which drains both legs and the pelvic abdominal areas and the left half of the upper body, including the head.
2. The right lymphatic duct, which drains the right half of the upper body and the head.

Spleen

The Spleen is the largest amount of lymphatic tissue in the body. It is responsible for storing and filtering old or damaged blood cells, plus bacteria, storing iron and the efficient re-use of the old cells to produce new haemoglobin. Its main function is to manufacture protective antibodies to fight off invaders, like bacteria or viruses. If it is removed by surgery (e.g. in a accident) the liver and bone marrow take over its functions.

Thymus

The Thymus gland monitors and regulates the energy flow of the body. Its function is not yet fully understood, thought it is known that it plays an important part in developing immunity against disease. It grows rapidly in young children because it is working hard to build immunity to disease and coping with the many illnesses of childhood. Their immune systems are not fully developed until about age twelve and the gland then shrinks after puberty. However, it still remains an important gland because it is involved in the production of T. Lymphocytes. These originate as white blood cells, which the lymphatic system has carried to the Thymus. There they multiply and are changed into special fighting cells, which are vital to the body's fight against tumour producing cells. Nowadays the role of the Thymus gland is being investigated in the immunological diseases like AIDS.

Located in the chest behind the breast bone and below the thyroid, the Thymus gland can be tapped externally, which is believed to stimulate the gland and boost the immune system.

Tonsils

The Tonsils, which are located at the back of the mouth and the adenoids, at the back of the nose, are also made up of lymphatic tissue. Their function is to act as special filters, especially in childhood. They are also involved in the formation of antibodies.

Reflexology and the Immune System:

- Reflexology stimulates the brain and opens the blocked energy pathways. If the immune system is blocked then nothing else will work properly. As a result the immune system will go down and the person is left open to infection and diseases.
- It helps to relax the body totally, thereby eliminating stress, which effects the immune system.
- It helps the body back into balance and normality. A relaxed and balanced body can then heal itself.
- The lymphatic system cleanses the body of toxins, so as Reflexology stimulates all the excretory organs, it is a very important aid in this cleansing process.
- The immune system deteriorates with age, so older people are more susceptible to infection and disease. Reflexology counteracts that by helping older people to feel better and it relieves their aches and pains.
- The constant companions of the elderly: impaired vision or hearing, stomach complaints, constipation and diarrhoea, arthritis, heart and bladder problems and diabetes, all respond well to this therapy. It also enhances the blood circulation, which then helps the brain and improve harmony.

THE CARDIOVASCULAR SYSTEM

The main components of the cardiovascular system are:

1) Heart
2) Lungs
3) Blood
4) Diaphragm

Blood is pumped from the heart to the lungs, where it receives fresh oxygen, it goes back to the heart to be pumped to all parts of the body. Arteries take the oxygen rich blood where it is needed and veins return the deoxygenated blood to the heart, to begin the process all over again. This system is powerfully affected by stress, leading to all kinds of problems including angina, heart attacks, high blood pressure, etc.

Heart

The heart is the most powerful muscle in the body. It is located in the chest cavity, one third on the right side of the central line and two thirds on the left side. It does an extraordinary amount of work, pumping 2,000 gallons of blood every twenty four hours.

The reflexes for the heart are on both feet, with two thirds situated on the left foot. Since the cardiovascular/circulatory system pertains to the whole body, it is vitally important to treat the whole body.

Lungs

The function of the lungs is to exchange the fresh oxygen (received by breathing) for the carbon dioxide brought to them in the blood, which they then get rid of by exhaling. This exchange takes place in tiny air sacs called alveoli. The lungs are one of the body's great eliminating systems, from the diaphragm up to the base of the neck, one on either side of the chest cavity. The lungs are protected by the ribs and covered by a membrane, the pleura, and when this becomes inflamed it is called pleurisy.

Blood

Blood is a specialized bodily fluid composed of blood cells suspended in a liquid called blood plasma, platelets and blood cells themselves. Plasma, which comprises 55% of blood fluid, is mostly water (90% by volume) and contains dissolved proteins, glucose, mineral ions, hormones, carbon dioxide (plasma being the main medium for excretory product transportation). The blood cells present in blood are mainly red blood cells and white blood cells, including leukocytes and platelets.

Diaphragm

The diaphragm is a strong sheet of muscle that divides the chest area from the area of the abdomen. It is the most important muscle for breathing. When it contracts the chest expands and we breathe in, when it relaxes the chest contracts and we breathe out. Relaxing the Diaphragm encourages better breathing. It is a key reflex for tension and stress and both feet are used in the treatment of asthma, bronchitis, pneumonia and emphysema.

Disorders of the Cardiovascular System: ANGINA

The heart retains about 5% of all the blood it pumps. This is fed into the heart muscle fibres by the coronary arteries, which surround the outside of the heart. If for any reason there is an inadequate supply of blood to the heart muscles there will be a lack of the vital oxygen and a spasm can occur. This is known as Angina Pectoris, a condition which affects both men and women in their middle to late years. People at risk are the ones with a family history, those who are overweight, who lead a sedentary life and people with a diet too high in saturated fats. Angina manifests as pain in the chest and also in the arms, neck, jaw and shoulders. Other facts which trigger angina are: cold weather, exercise after a heavy meal, emotional upsets, hypertension due to stress, etc.

Reflexology and the Cardiovascular System

To help relieve acute angina pain grasp the tip of the little finger of your left hand (the area above the first joint) with your right thumb and forefinger and hold it tightly. Grasping the little toe in the same way also helps, then work on the heart reflex area in either your left hand or left foot. This is located on the sole of the left foot between the diaphragm line and the base of the toes. Work the entire area, thumb walking up, down and across, take your time and work this area thoroughly. You can also work on the corresponding areas on the palm of your left and right hands.

Recommendations:

- Diet, reduce fat and salt intake, avoid junk foods, eat more fresh fruit and vegetables.
- Stop smoking.
- Have regular gentle exercise: 20 minute walk, gentle yoga, tai-chi, climb several flights of stairs.
- Keep a check on cholesterol levels and blood pressure.
- Reduce tension.

The circulation of the blood is extremely important to the proper functioning of the heart and this is where reflexology helps as:

- It improves the circulation all over the body.
- It helps muscular function.
- It balances blood pressure by reducing stress and tension.
- It relieves aches and pains and will keep arthritis at bay.
- It helps with digestion and to clear the body of toxins.
- The circulation is improved, giving warmth to hands and feet.
- It reduces stress.
- The healing touch offered on a one to one basis helps to balance the indifference of the family and the world.
- It helps to overcome the sense of helplessness and hopelessness and reduces the sense of loneliness.
- It balances the whole body, helping the person to feel better about themselves and their health.
- Bladder problems, oedema and constipation is helped.
- A state of deep natural relaxation is induced and sleep quality is greatly improved.

THE RESPIRATORY SYSTEM

It is the complicated system by which we breathe and is the area most susceptible to allergies and infections. The main components of the respiratory system are:

1) Nose and Throat
2) Trachea
3) Sinuses
4) Lungs
5) Diaphragm

Nose and Throat

The air cleaning system starts in the nose, throat and bronchial tubes, where tiny hairs move backwards and forwards to trap foreign particles going any further.

These tiny hairs are paralysed by smoking, they can die and the foreign bodies can then plug the vital air sacs into each lungs, resulting in emphysema and other diseases.

Trachea

The trachea, or windpipe, is the vertical tube extending down from the larynx to immediately above the heart, where it divides into two main bronchi, one extending to each lung.

Sinuses

The sinuses are air filled spaces in the cheekbones and behind the eyebrows, which are linked to the nose. They have mucus glands and tiny hairs which convey the mucus into the nasal cavity. These mucus membranes can become infected in colds, flu and sinusitis, which can become chronic.

Lungs (see Cardiovascular System)

Diaphragm (see Cardiovascular System)

Disorders of the Respiratory System: ASTHMA

The conditions which affect the respiratory system e.g. bronchitis, asthma, emphysema, are known to respond well to Reflexology. Asthma is, particularly in children, very much on the increase and is a particularly distressing condition, both to the patient and the family. There are many reasons for this increase like: the additives in both food and drink, the increasing pollution of the atmosphere, problems with allergens (dust mites from fitted carpets, double glazing and central heating), sprays of all kinds, used in the home and in the countryside, stress of any kind, pet hairs that irritate the nostrils and the mucus membranes of the nose and lungs, chemicals, medicines, processed food, etc.

Reflexology helps to increase the capacity of the lungs by stimulating the diaphragm to contract and relax fully. Children respond very well to this treatment, with a consequent reduction in their wheezing. This may lead them to want to discard inhalers or stop medication. This should not be encouraged without the doctor's consent. Self help aids for them should include: deep breathing exercises, swimming, playing a wind instrument, exercise (e.g. running or brisk walking).

THE DIGESTIVE SYSTEM

The Digestive System (also known as the alimentary canal) is the system of organs, within multi cellular animals, that takes in food, digests it to extract energy and nutrients and expels the remaining waste. The major functions of the digestive system are: ingestion, digestion, absorption and defecation.

The main components of the digestive system are:

1) Upper gastrointestinal tract:
   Mouth
   Pharynx
   Esophagus
   Stomach

2) Lower gastrointestinal tract:
   Small intestine (Duodenum, Jejunum, Ileum)
   Large intestine (Cecum, Colon, Rectum)
   Anus

3) Accessory organs:
   Liver (employing the gallbladder as a reservoir)
   Pancreas

Upper Gastrointestinal Tract:

Mouth

The mouth (or oral cavity) is the first portion of the alimentary canal that receives food and begins digestion by mechanically breaking up the solid food particles into smaller pieces and mixing them with saliva. Food provides us with:

- Fuel to live.
- Energy to work and play.
- The raw materials with which to build new cells.

Pharynx

It is part of the digestive system and respiratory system of many organisms. Because both food and air pass through the pharynx, a flap of connective tissue, called the epiglottis, closes over the trachea when food is swallowed to prevent choking or aspiration. In humans the pharynx is important in vocalization.

Esophagus

The esophagus, sometimes known as the gullet, is an organ in vertebrates which consists of a muscular tube through which food passes from the pharynx to the stomach.

Stomach

As the food comes into the muscular sac, which is the stomach, wave-like muscular contractions sweep from top to bottom, mixing the food with the gastric juices into a thin mash and moving it on down towards the intestines.

Lower Gastrointestinal Tract:

Small Intestine

The small intestine plays a major role in digestion and absorption of nutrients from food. It is a tube 6-7 metres long which doubles back on itself. After absorption it pushes the foot along towards the colon.

Large Intestine

It consists of the ascending, transverse and descending colon. The digestion of food is now complete and absorption is the main function of the Large Intestine. It absorbs water and salts in order to conserve the body fluids.

Anus

The anus is an opening at the opposite end of the digestive tract from the mouth. Its function is to expel faeces. One of the most common problems that can affect the area of the anus are the haemorrhoids. The basic treatment for haemorrhoids is the same as the best preventative measure: a diet rich in fibre from fresh fruit, vegetables and bran. Reflexology has been found to be very good for haemorrhoids: working up the back of the heel will bring great relief, giving this area special attention, expecially on the sides, where there will be a lot of tightening and pain.

Accessory Organs:

Liver

One of the organs associated with the digestive system, the liver, is one of the most powerful and important organs of the body. It weights 3lbs and is mostly on the right hand side below the diaphragm. It stores vitamins, iron, copper, glycogen and bile. It is a very powerful detox agent and cleans the intestinal blood. It manufactures bile and cholesterols, enzymes and blood coagulation factors and can regenerate itself. It maintains blood sugar levels.

The Gall Bladder: is embedded in the liver, about ½ way between the waistline and diaphragm (zones 3-4). The main function is to store the bile which has been produced by the liver, releasing it as needed to emulsify fats.

Pancreas

Its juices are essential for the digestion of proteins, fats and carbohydrates. It helps to neutralise the acidity of the stomach juices and, working with the liver, it maintains blood sugar levels.

Disorders of the Digestive System: HIATUS HERNIA

When food is swallowed it passes through the oesophagus to the stomach. If there is a weakness or a spasm at the point where the oesophagus passes through the diaphragm, at the neck of the stomach, the stomach can bulge through, which then leads to a certain amount of re-flux of the stomach's contents upwards.

As this contains stomach acids, any re-flux will aggravate the lining of the oesophagus, making it sore and giving rise to symptoms as:

- Pain.
- Indigestion.
- Anxiety attacks.
- A lump in the throat.
- An inability to gain weight.

If the stomach gets caught the hernia can become strangulated, trapping the blood supply. This can cause acute pain, which is relieved only by surgery. Some of the symptoms are often confused with those of a heart attack. To alleviate the symptoms:

- Remain upright immediately after a meal.
- Avoid large meals, especially before bedtime. Frequent smaller meals are better than three large ones.
- Avoid tightly-waisted clothes, which squeeze the upper abdomen.
- Raise the head of the bed for greater comfort when sleeping.

Aloe Vera juice (mixed with fruit juice) is reputed to soothe and heal the lining of the oesophagus. It works by blocking the inflammatory agents which could cause pain or inflammation.

Emotionally speaking, worry affects the stomach adversely, people who are worriers then will suffer stomach ailments most.

Many of the elderly will suffer some form of Hiatus Hernia, especially women. Working on the feet correspondent to the diaphragm/solar plexus area will result in relaxation of the muscles and a relief of tension, which is why Reflexology can help greatly in this condition.

THE URINARY SYSTEM

The Urinary System is the organ system that produces, stores and eliminate urine. The two kidneys, two ureters, the bladder and the urethra filter the blood and, in co-operation with the sweat glands, they control the salt and water content of the body. They also get rid of toxic waste in the urine, which is 96% water and 4% uric acid, urea and salts. The system also maintains the balance between acid and base and is extremely important to the Reflexologist because elimination of toxins is vital for the maintenance of balance in the body, with resultant well-being. The main components of the urinary system are:

1) Kidneys
2) Ureters
3) Bladder
4) Urethra

Kidneys

The kidneys are two of the master organs in the body. They consist of millions of nephrons which make up one of the most efficient filtering systems known to man. They have a capacity of a staggering 1300 litres a day. They are located, one on either side of the body, in the lower back and are important to remember when kidney stones, oedema and gout are present and also when non urinary diseases, like high blood pressure, affects the body. The kidney reflex is found in the centre of the foot, above and below the waistline. By stimulating it the filter process is helped to maximise its potential.

Ureters

The urethras are very thin tubes which carry the urine from the kidneys to the bladder. Blockages (e.g. stones) may occur here. The ureter reflexes are from the kidneys down to the bladder.

Bladder

The bladder is a balloon shaped sac, which stores up to a pint of urine until it is expelled. When infected the reflex area can be red and puffy. The infection can easily block the ureter tubes to the kidneys, which makes it far more serious. The bladder reflex is on the inside edge of both feet and below the heel guideline, next to the lower part of the spine reflex.

Urethra

The urethra is a tube which connects the urinary bladder to the outside of the body. The urethra has an excretory function in both sexes to pass urine to the outside and also a reproductive function in the male, as a passage for semen.

Disorders of the Urinary System: CYSTITIS

Cystitis is an inflammation of the lining of the bladder. It is especially common in women because the pathway to invasion by infecting bacteria is helped by a shorter urethra (4 cm as against 20 cm in men); because of the proximity of the urethra to the anus and the penetration of organisms following intercourse. Cystitis should never be taken lightly, as the infection can easily block the tubes to the kidneys, leading to serious illness. Ignoring the body's urges to urinate weakens the bladder by stretching it unnecessarily, resulting in stagnation of the urine, leading to further bladder infections. Infection often occurs due to stress or when the organism is run down. Recurrent cystitis can also be troublesome after the menopause due to a lack of oestrogen, which causes the skin to thin in this area. The Symptoms are:

- The hypersensitivity of the nerve endings in the bladder wall, caused by the inflammation, leads to a incresing desire to urinate frequently.
- A sharp pain on passing water and low pelvic pain.
- Foul smelling urine, which may contain pus.

- Blood in the urine when a severe infection occurs.
- The whole body feels unwell and shivery .
- Oedema (fluid retention) in hands and under the eyes.

Prevention:

- Drink at least eight glasses of water per day or more.
- Avoid coffee, tea and alcohol, which dehydrates the system.
- Urinate when the need arises and empty the bladder completely without rushing.
- Wash the genital area (from front to back) morning and evening.
- Avoid bubble bath, perfumed soaps, bath gels, deodorant, talc or antiseptics on genital area. Try and use "simple" soap.
- Have a shower instead of a bath.
- Use all cotton underwear next to the skin.
- Avoid tight jeans, nylon panties or tights (except especially designed ones).
- Use a non petroleum based lubricating jelly to prevent soreness and bruising on intercourse.
- After intercourse (10 minutes) pass water.
- After a bowel movement, scrupulous hygiene in the washing of the hands and nails, plus a sluice down (from front to back) is essential. With frequent or chronic cystitis it is necessary to wash the penis and the genital area before intercourse with water only (preferably boiled which is allowed to cool before use).
- When the infection has passed drinking cranberry juice helps to prevent further attacks.

Reflexology helps to stimulate the urinary system to heal itself. It helps with the oedema by releasing the water held on to by the body. The toxins are released plus the residue from dormant previous infections. It helps to alleviate the pain.

Disorder of the Urinary System: I. B. S.

Irritable Bowel Syndrome (I.B.S.) is an increasingly common ailment of the digestive tract. Stress and tension are associated with it and continuing stress aggravates it. Women are more susceptible to this complain than men. The two main symptoms are abdominal pain and altered bowel habits, which tend to move erratically from diarrhoea to constipation, plus a bloated abdomen due to excessive wind. The pain is usually relieved after a bowel movement or on passing wind. A sensation that the bowel is incompletely emptied is particularly distressing. Sufferers are usually hard striving perfectionists who find it difficult to relax. Research in the U. S. A. has shown that the intestine has a much greater influence on the brain and the entire personality than hitherto thought. Local irritation of the bowel usually reflects the irritation of the whole person, whether they realise it or not. Emotional problems have been shown to have a negative effect on the bacterial flora of the intestine. In I.B.S. there is usually a problem in the emotional field, in the inability to cope with an inflammatory situation.

Food is said to be responsible for at least 1/3 of the cases. Some people find that the condition can trigger duodenal or stomach ulcers. It can cause weight loss, poor health and frequent bowel movements can cause haemorrhoids. The physical symptoms are often accompanied by fatigue, depression and anxiety. It is very important to look at the diet to make nutritional changes.

Avoid: cows milk and diary products, coffee, alcohol, bran, onions, beans, peas, lentils, cabbage and broccoli.

Eat: fish, chicken, root vegetables, rice, pasta, potatoes, pears, stewed apples, balanced duet of fresh vegetables, fruit and rice.

Eat several small meals per day instead of 3 large ones. Try to pinpoint the stress, lifestyle or food which is causing it or triggering off an attack. Lack of exercise adds to this problem. The stomach and liver reflexes will be sensitive due to digestive imbalance. The small intestine or the colon, especially the sigmoid, will be extremely sensitive, or the anus and rectum if haemorrhoids are present. Apart from irritable bowel the patient may have a lot of pain in the neck and shoulders. Perfectionists with a lot of responsibility tend to "carry the world on their shoulders".

The lower back may also be involved as there are nerves there which connect to the colon. Reflexology helps irritable bowel syndrome by reducing tension and abdominal bloating.

Disorder of the Urinary System: MENSTRUAL PROBLEMS

- Disturbances, pain at ovulation time.
- Period pains, hot flushes.
- Barrenness.
- Cysts.

How can reflexology help:

- People will say their hot flushes have lessened.
- Their moods are not erratic.
- They are more relaxed.
- Less disturbance with premenstrual problems.

THE SKELETAL SYSTEM

The Skeletal system is not just a collection of bones, it is instead quite astonishing in its complexity and in the range of its functions. It provides a framework for the body, thereby giving us a shape. In providing this frame the skeleton protects the vital organs:

- The skull protects the brain.
- The rib-cage protects the heart and lungs.
- The spinal column protects the spinal cord.
- The pelvic bones protect the organs in the abdominal area.

Bones

The skeletal system consists of 206 bones, ¼ of which are in the feet, 26 in each foot and 28 in each hand. Together the hands and feet contain more than one half of the bones of the entire body. In each foot there are 26 bones, 107 ligaments and 19 muscles supporting and balancing the rest of the body. If the feet are out of alignment the whole structure suffers.

The tarsal bones can be compared to the wrist bones. The 5 metatarsals (long bones) compare to the metacarpals of the hand. The 14 phalanges of the toes correspond to the phalanges of the fingers and thumbs.

There are 5 types of bones:

1) Long (e.g. the femur).
2) Short (e.g. the metatarsals in the feet).
3) Flat (e.g. the frontal bones in the head).
4) Irregular (e.g. the vertebra in the spine).
5) Sesamoid or rounded (e.g. the knee cap).

Whereas the bones have a huge role in supporting the body and in protecting the organs, they are also chemical factories involved in the production of the components of the blood, minerals and other vital constituents. Then too they act as a reservoir for most of the body's needs, including 99% of the calcium, 88% of the phosphorus, as well as copper and cobalt. The calcium is released as required and plays a very important role in maintaining a delicate balance in the body. Most of the replacements of the red blood cells are provided for by the bones, an enormous task considering the blood utilises 180 million red blood cells every minute. Every day red and white cells, bone marrow, as well as platelet cells are all manufactured in the bones. In addition they also contain millions of osteoblast cells which produce collagen, a protein which forms the beginning of new bone, which is constantly needed as replacement, all over the body.

Reflexology can help the conditions like: arthritis, osteoporosis, kyphosis, gout, scoliosis, lordois, bunions, ankylosis, etc.

• By increasing circulation to the joints, Reflexology helps
  to break down the uric acid, calcium and other deposits, which

may have lodged there. This helps to prevent or modify diseases (e.g. gout) which are caused by such deposits.

- By stimulating better blood flow to knees, elbows, shoulders, etc. Reflexology helps these areas to remain supple. By increasing the flexibility it prevents stiffness setting in, especially when the person is inactive.

- Reflexology releases tension, which eases rigidity and loosens the muscles. This relaxes the frame and frees up movement.

- Reflexology is a great help to a person having chiropractic treatment. By releasing tension the muscles of the back are relaxed, thereby helping to increase the benefit from the chiropractic adjustments.

- Athletes too are greatly helped by a reflexology treatment. When receiving regular treatment not only are their bodies more in balance, but it has been found that they are less prone to injury. It has also been noted that when injured, their recovery is quicker and more complete.

- Reflexology helps to reduce swelling around the ankles and knees, this frees up movement.

- Reflexology helps to speed up healing after fractures etc. or post operatively.

The bones of the foot are of great interest to the reflexologist and can be compared to the bones of the hand:

Metatarsals bones of foot - metacarpals of hand.
Tarsal bones of foot - carpals of hand.

This similarity can be used to great advantage if, for whatever reason, Reflexology cannot be use on the feet, it can be used instead on the hands. This is especially helpful where painful skeletal ailments like arthritis are concerned. Importantly the bones act as lever for the muscles and so they facilitate movement.

When the muscles move they move the bones and so we walk, bend, run, etc.

Bones are connected to each other by joints, there are 3 types:

- <u>Fixed</u> or immovable (e.g. the skull bones).
- <u>Slightly movable</u> (e.g. the sacroiliac joint in the pelvis).
- <u>Freely movable.</u> These joints are in a fibrous capsule, which is lined with synovial membrane and contains synovial fluid in the cavity to reduce friction between the surfaces of the joint. This cavity is called a bursa and when it becomes inflames it thickens. This is what happens when a bunion is formed, the joint enlarges and can then displace the toe or make it crooked.

Crystals of uric acid can build up in the joints, so the kidneys need to be flushed out constantly and regularly to prevent this.

To maintain healthy bones vitamin D is essential in the diet, plus adequate amounts of calcium, vitamins and proteins. The skeletal system needs a constant blood supply to help muscles and nerves to function well.

<u>Spine</u>

The spine is in the centre of the body's equilibrium. It is strong yet flexible and supports the head as well as giving attachment to the ribs. It is required daily to bend, twist and contort itself and is put under more stress than virtually any other bone structure in the body, which can lead to innumerable problems. It is a fantastic structure and is designed and curved in such a way as to absorb the daily shocks of walking, lifting, running, bending, etc.

It contains 33 bones, 24 of which are movable vertebrae, separated by pads or discs of fibro cartilage that allow the vertebrae to move without friction. Injury to or loss of one of these discs is the basis for much pain and discomfort.

The bones of the spine support the trunk of the body, provide secure anchorage for the muscles in the back and protects the spinal cord, the vital lifeline to the rest of the body, with its vast supply of nerves that radiate out from there. The structure of the spine closely follows the structure of the foot. The adult spine has 4 curves as has each foot and the spine has 26 vertebrae while the foot has 26 bones.

Rib Cage

The rib cage has 12 pairs of ribs. These are connected to the spine at the back and to the sternum or breast bone at the front. The ribs protect the heart and the lungs. There are:

7 pairs of true ribs which are connected to both front and back.

3 pairs of false ribs which are directly connected to the back and indirectly to the front.

2 pairs of floating ribs which are only connected to the back.

THE ENDOCRINE SYSTEM

The endocrine glands, secreting hormones, are responsible for controlling the complex activities of the body, especially all the changes that occurs in it. The hormones are the messengers of the endocrine system, they are responsible for transmitting the vital informations directly into the blood stream.

The main components of the endocrine system are:

1) Pituitary Gland
2) Adrenal Glands
3) Thyroid
4) Parathyroids
5) Pancreas
6) Reproductive Glands

Pituitary Gland

The pituitary gland is located at the base of the brain and produces several hormones that perform different functions:

a) Growth (structural and soft tissue growth)
b) Metabolism (supervising cells work)
c) Regulation (regulate the other endocrine glands, blood supply, water balance, blood pressure, sexual functions, temperature)

Adrenal Glands

The adrenal glands are located on top of each kidneys and have many functions that interrelate with the other glands. The adrenals secrete hormones which control the balance of water and minerals and maintain the muscle tone to promote a healthy digestion. They reduce inflammation, prevent excessive stress and fight fatigue.

The Adrenaline is a hormone that stimulate blood pressure and circulation in heart and mussels and prepares the body for action during an emergency situation (fear), meanwhile it releases glucose, stimulate breathing and slow down digestive and excretive processes.

Thyroid

The tyroid gland is located in the front of the neck and regulates the metabolism of the cells of the body.

Some hormones effect bone growth, control calcium levels, while others control skin health and cholesterol level.

Treating the tyroid is therefore good for high cholesterol and sluggish metabolism. With an over-active thyroid a person could be restless, nervous, irritable, tired, have weight loss, etc.

Parathyroids

The parathyroids are 4 glands embedded in the thyroid. Their hormones control the levels of calcium and phosphorous in the blood. This is very important because keeps the skeletal system in order as well as nerve and muscle tissue, preventing kidney stones, nervous conditions, arthritis, cramps and weak muscles.

Pancreas

The pancreas lies behind the stomach. It has both endocrine and exocrine function, respectively secreting hormones into the bloodstream and secreting juices through the pancreatic duct, to neutralize acid from the stomach and producing enzymes that break down complex substances. The hormone insulin is essential for the control of the glucose level in the blood, a failure to supply enough insulin causes diabetes and an over production of insulin (hypoglycemia) can impair the efficiency of the brain.

Reproductive Glands

The reproductive glands are located in correspondence of the sexual organs. The sex hormones influence the reproductive capacity, maintain sexual urge, mental vigour and physical development. They are used also by the adrenal glands and vice versa.

FOURTH SECTION

1. Quick Tips for Happy Feet

2. Relaxation Techniques

3. Self Help to Well Being

4. Health & Fitness

5. Reflexology is my Little Treat

6. Listening

7. Preventative Therapy

8. What your feet can tell you about your health

9. Being positive about your thinking

10. Female & Male Menopause

11. Responsibility for our own health

12. Old Cures from the past

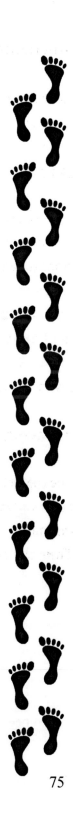

QUICK TIPS FOR HAPPY FEET

When feet are tired the whole body is tired. Feet are very often neglected and abused, which can be reflected in the face. It would pay dividends to pamper them now and then and feel the relaxing effects throughout the body. Stand in cold water up to the ankles. This relaxes the feet and enhances sleep. Cool down hot feet with a mint, cypress, aloe vera or tea tree gel rub; these are cooling and reviving gels which revitalise heavy legs or tired feet, soothe and refresh swollen ankles and improve the circulation. A vegetable oil spiked with clove oil when rubbed into the feet will soothe and revitalise them. The best base oils for this include avocado, olive and sesame. A good soak in warm water before bedtime benefits the feet greatly, when hard skin can be removed more easily and a good oil or cream e.g. calendula, witch hazel or mint can be rubbed in to finish. Always make sure to dry thoroughly in between the toes after bathing or showering. Never neglect corns, athlete's foot, verruca, etc. Seek professional advice sooner rather than later. Ill-fitting shoes result in corns, calluses and bunions, which develop from the repeated rubbing or pressure. Shoes should be changed regularly during the day, especially from high heels to flat ones for continuous wear. It is not recommended to wear the same shoes day after day. A change of footwear is good both for the wearer and for the shoes. Women are more prone to these complaints because of the shoes they wear, rather than men who in general have good feet. Foot exercise: with the sole of the foot roll a golf ball lightly from toe to heel, this exercises all the foot and relaxes it.

RELAXATION TECHNIQUES

Since one of the main goals of Reflexology is to reduce stress in the body, these relaxation techniques are used throughout a full treatment at various times, especially if the client is tense and anxious. But they are especially beneficial at the end of a programme, leaving the client with a wonderfully relaxed feeling of well being.

Foot shaking:
The hands are placed on either side of the foot and with a vigorous movement the foot is lightly slapped backwards and forwards with a loose flowing movement. This helps the circulation, eases tenderness and relaxes the muscles in the ankle and calf.

Ankle loosening:
Using the heel of the palms, the hands are moved rapidly backwards and forwards over the ankles to encourage the circulation.

Ankle rotation:
While holding the heel of the foot in the palm of one hand, the top of the foot is firmly held with the other hand and the foot is then smoothly rotated, first in one direction and then in the other direction a number of times. It is then pulled forward and stretched backwards gently. This stretches the Achilles tendon.

Ankle massage:
Both thumbs are used here to massage the ankle area, in an outward movement from the centre of the foot, the rest of the hand acts as support.

Toe rotation:

This is similar to ankle rotation, as both loosen the joints. The thumb and fingers are used with the fingers extending right down over the toes. The toes are then rotated, first in one direction and equally in the opposite direction with a slight upward pull. This movement is very good for relaxing tension in the neck.

Toe stretching:

Each toe is stretched backwards and forwards with good support. The toes are also loosened from the bottom to the top, using quick stroking movements of all fingers.

Spinal Massaging and stretching:

The inside of the foot along the spinal areas is gently stroked and massaged using the full palm, with light circular movements from top to bottom of the area.

Spinal twist:

The hands are placed around the foot with the thumbs together on the sole at the arch and all 8 fingers together on the top. One hand is turned, while keeping the other stationary, in a wringing twisting movement, which is started at the lower area and worked upwards towards the toes.

Diaphragm rocking:

This technique is used midway through treatment when the client is very relaxed. Both thumbs are placed under the diaphragm reflex and meeting at the solar plexus point. The 4 fingers are together on the top of the foot with the index fingers touching and forming a "V" towards the ankles. The foot is then rocked gently back and forth, pressing on the solar plexus reflex while going forward and stretching the metatarsal bones on the top of the foot as it rocks back. This is deeply relaxing for the client and is done about 15 times on each foot, or more if the client is deeply anxious.

Kneading:

The back of the fingers, between the knuckles of the practitioners hand, are used here on the sole of the foot. Starting at the base of the toes and working slowly downwards in a rotating movement, the area is kneaded with a light touch. This is a very soothing technique used to ventilate the chest and lung areas.

Heel kneading:

While supporting the foot in the palm of one hand, the heel is kneaded (as you would dough) for the sciatic and pelvic areas. Continuing with the thumb and fingers, beginning at the ankle bone at the top of the heel, the achilles tendon and lower calf muscles are massaged gently upwards.

Feathering:

Here, the fingers are run repeatedly down the toes, top and sides of the foot from toes to ankle and back again in long sweeping movements, with a feathery touch. Then very gently and lightly the toes are feathered upwards repeatedly. This relaxed the client, inducing a luxurious feeling of pampering.

Thumb stroking:
The sole and sides of the foot are worked here using a criss-cross movement of the thumbs, while keep them parallel to each other. This massages and stretches the sole. Then very lightly and gently the thumbs are drawn slowly over the top from ankle to ankle (used towards the end).

Solar plexus deep breathing:
The solar plexus area stores anxiety and tension. It is a barometer of emotional well-being. This technique, which is generally used at the end of a session, helps the client to release any lingering bit of stress and is deeply relaxing. The thumbs of both hands are placed on the reflex and, while firm pressure is applied, the client takes in a deep breath, holds it as the feet are lifted up and breathes out as the pressure is released. This is generally repeated three times.

SELF HELP TO WELL BEING

You can do Reflexology on yourself by working on the hand:

For constipation:
With four fingers together, pull down and across the heel of the thumb to the wrist.

For eyes and ears:
For the outer ear: using 1st finger and thumb press into the web between the small finger and the next finger.
For the inner ear: press between the 2nd and 3rd fingers.

For the eyes:
Press between the 1st and 2nd fingers.

For headache:
Work the top of the thumb up and down from base to nail bed.

For kidneys:
To get rid of excess uric acid work down from the 2nd and 3rd fingers and about 2" from the wrist, press in and up on both hands.

For hair growth:
Buffing the nails together briskly for 5 minutes, 3-4 times a day.

For immune system:
One hand, palm down, is placed on the chest bone midway between the breasts with the 2nd hand over it. This stimulates the pineal gland.

For infection:
The adrenal gland (on the top of the kidneys) can be stimulated by using the same method as for the kidneys, on both hands.

For mucus:
On the palm of the right hand, down from the web between the small and the next fingers, press in for the illeocecal valve.

For nervous tension:
Clasp the hands tightly together as in prayer and release.

For pituitary and hormonal balance:
Press the centre of the widest part of the underside of the thumb in and up, both hands.

For sinus trouble:
Using the fleshy tips of both thumbs press in and upwards under the bones of the eyebrows. Hold for 1-2 seconds.

For sinus drainage:
Using the soft tips of the 3rd finger on both hands, work in a very light stroking movement across the check bone from the bridge of the nose to the outer edge of the face. To free blockages use an inward rotating movement on the side of the nose.

For sleep:
Shine a torch on the spot midway between the eyes on the forehead, which is the site of the third eye. This will also enhance the mood of S. A. D. sufferers.

To stimulate the whole body:
Hold the rolled flaps at the top of the ears with 2 fingers and a thumb and roll outwards, while moving slowly down to the end of the ears.

HEALTH AND FITNESS

Things you should know about your feet:
Your feet will carry you about 70,000 miles in a lifetime. They

contain 29 bones, 19 muscles, 115 ligaments and about 250,000 sweat glands each. Sweat is odourless, but if bacteria is present it creates an unpleasant smell. Feet need to be washed regularly.

When the feet get hot and clammy they are susceptible to athlete's foot, which is a fungal infection that can be passed around in gyms and swimming pools if care is not taken. Flip-flops need to be used. Socks need to be washed separately to stop this fungal infection spreading to other people. Verruca is another thing to watch out for. One should seek help from a chiropodist, make sure they are registered. If you look after your feet, they will look after your body.

REFLEXOLOGY IS MY LITTLE TREAT

Most women like to get their hair washed and blow-dried regularly, which makes us feel good and look good. Why not give our feet a treat now and then? When one's feet are tired, the rest of our bodies feel the same. If we feel good after having our hair done, what would it be like after having pampered our feet? After all, we spend a lot of money on make up for our faces. Our feet do so much looking after our whole bodies, its time now to look after our feet. Think about it and look for a good reflexologist in your area. It will serve you well. Look after your feet and they will look after you. I thought I would share this little secret with you: one evening I was sitting in my room, had a bad headache wondering how I would get rid of it. As I looked around the room my eyes glanced at two golf balls, I started to think, remembering hearing about someone using a golf ball on their hands and thought I would give it a try. I got the golf ball down on the floor and worked my feet up and down, one at a time. After ten minutes, to my amazement my headache had disappeared. So simple yet so effective. You know what to do now when you are feeling below par, get a golf ball, it will do the trick.

LISTENING

Listening to what is being said is a wonderful art to have. Sometimes we think we are listening, but are we or are we not hearing what is really being said? Do we just hear words and not what lies behind what the person is really saying?

When we listen there are three things involved:

• Words
• Tone
• Non-verbal communication

Tone sometimes says something different from the words used. Tone and non verbal really speak the message. There are obstacles to listening which are coming from internal and external sources, which causes conflict and blocks us from listening and not hearing what is being said. A good listener is a treasure.

As reflexologists we are trained to listen to what the clients are saying, also listening to what the feet are communicating to us and what they are showing to the therapist.

PREVENTATIVE THERAPY

Health care has become a top priority for many in today's world. Many pay frequent and often unnecessary visits to the doctor's surgery, taking away with them prescriptions for health promoting tablets and capsules. In recent years however there is a growing awareness of the truth that there are other methods of preserving and promoting good health. Acupuncture, aroma therapy and reflexology are just three of them. These therapies are not to be seen as either opposed to conventional medicine or a substitute for it. Many health disorders can be both diagnosed and dealt with by these complimentary therapies, thus leaving the doctor free to deal with health disorders which require his or her expert professional skill.

Reflexology has a well established reputation as an effective means of both discovering health disorders and also dealing with them. Complementary Therapy can prove very beneficial if it is approached with openness and a positive attitude. For the body to be healthy everything must work together, therefore it is essential to have it "tuned up" with all the parts running smoothly and what better way than to avail of a reflexology treatment. This therapy brings peace and relaxation to the body, calms the mind and restores mental alertness.

My personal belief is that Reflexology can be a wonderful means of relaxation and gives a feeling of well being. It can ward off illness and fatigue and enhances everyday life. People are becoming more conscious of their health and surely there is nothing better than the truly holistic approach, where mind, body and emotions are interwoven, allowing us to function to our full capacity.

Giving the environment we are living in, today our health is threatened. Our polluted land, air and water, contaminated food, stress of day to day living, etc. are lethal to attract disease.

Most people wait until they get ill before seeking help. We look after our cars, not realising that our bodies need care to maintain balance within our systems. We need physical, emotional and spiritual healing. We need to recognise that there is harmony between these three elements working well together, one cannot work without the other. It would serve one well to have some sort of preventative therapy from time to time.

I will list a few of these therapies which may suit:

- Reflexology
  Using the meridians and minor chakra points, by massaging certain points on the hands or feet, therapeutic effects are assumed for the internal organs and other parts of the body that are connected to these points via the nervous system.

- Massage
  The systematic therapeutic stroking or kneading of the body or part of it. The manipulation of the soft tissues of the body in order to reduce tension and stress, increase circulation, aid the healing of muscle and other soft-tissue injuries, control pain and promote overall well-being.

- Meditation
  The practice of sitting or resting quietly and performing mental exercises designed to relax the body and focus concentration.

Glossary of other Healing Methods:

Acupuncture

In China and neighboring countries, acupuncture has been practiced for 6,000 years. It consists of the use of very fine needles and other devices to stimulate and balance the flow of energy, known as chi or qi, through channels or meridians in the body. Disease occurs because of imbalances in the meridian system.

Acupuncture is based on ancient Chinese ideas about the rhythm and harmony of the universe as a whole, the Tao and the relationship of human beings to that universe. Health is viewed as a dynamic interaction between each individual's inner environment and the exterior world.

Alexander Technique

The Alexander Technique is concerned with the mechanics of coordination and balance and our control over them. These things begin to deteriorate in most of us quite early in childhood and the process continues as the stresses of modern life take their toll. Excessive effort and tension become insidiously ingrained in our habits of movement, thought and feeling. Through an increase in muscular tensions we may notice this deterioration in neck, back, legs and wrists. The Alexander Technique aims to help you take a fresh look at the way you think and move, in everyday activities as well as specific skills.

Aromatherapy

Aromatherapy employs highly concentrated essential oils extracted from herbs and flowers that contain hormones, vitamins, antibiotics, and antiseptics. Applied to the skin, often in massage or through inhalation, the oil or combination of oils can be used for medicinal, meditative, restorative, or relaxation purposes.

Astrology

Astrology uses a birth chart to map the positions of the planets relative to the location and moment of birth. The interpretation of the chart incorporates the angular relationships between the planets and the signs of the zodiac, the area of the chart in which they fall and other symbolic indicators to examine the different experiences and psychology of the individual. A trained astrologer then analyzes the pertinent information, exploring how the various aspects of the client's personality may be integrated and finding ways to draw the greatest fulfillment from the energies symbolized in the chart.

Avatar

Avatar is a powerful and speedily effective course based on the simple truth that your beliefs will cause you to create or attract situations and events that you experience as your life. Explore your own belief system with the tools to modify things that you wish to change.

Ayurveda

The Sanskrit word meaning "science of life," Ayurveda is Yoga's sister science, dating back to the ancient Vedic civilization, the oldest tradition of knowledge in human history. Ayurveda is not a modality, but a comprehensive body of knowledge based upon the observation of living beings and their environment, appreciation of the balance between the individual and the cosmos and how to maintain balance and develop the consciousness that underlies and integrates all aspects of life, leading to self-realization, the goal it shares with Yoga.

Ayurveda does this through its insight into the various body/mind constitutions, called Prakriti, which is the innate balance of three primary principles or energies, called Doshas. Health is defined as the maintenance of balance among the Doshas according to one's unique constitution. Its methodologies include, but are not limited to: nutrition, herbalism, aromatherapy, yoga asana, meditation and bodywork.

Bau Biologie

Bau Biologie is the study of the biological and ecological aspects of living in buildings, and provides methods for detecting and eliminating sources of environmental pollution and sick building syndrome that cause biological stress and contribute to ill health and disease. This includes harmful electrical and magnetic radiation, indoor air and water pollution, molds and toxic building materials.

Bodytalk

Since most illnesses have a number of contributing factors, from hormones to stress, physical trauma, environmental toxins and nutrition, it's often difficult to know where to begin the healing process. Fortunately every person has an Innate Wisdom within them that knows exactly what they need to heal on all levels.

Bodytalk is a simple, effective method of communicating with that Innate Wisdom to discover the level each person needs to heal first.

Once the priority for healing has been discovered, a gentle tapping is used to re-harmonize the neglected area. It is astonishing how quickly the body and mind can heal once we allow it to communicate better within itself and with us. All we have to do is ask.

Bradley Method

Based on the philosophies of the late Dr. Robert Bradley, the pioneering obstetrician who first invited fathers into the delivery room 50 years ago, the Bradley Method is the most successful natural childbirth method today. In a comprehensive 8 to 12 week Bradley course, expectant parents learn to make educated choices and are given the tools they need to experience a natural, unmedicated birth.

Chiropractic

Chiropractic care employs gentle and forceful manipulation and movement techniques to correct spinal-nerve interferences. It removes blockages to the flow of Life Energy from the brain down the spinal cord, through the nervous system and out to every cell. Chiropractors assist in maintaining the body's natural alignment so that it functions at peak performance. They have been successful in treating headaches, back problems and other traumas.

Coaching

Coaching is a relationship in which the client and the coach are active collaborators for the purpose of meeting the client's needs. The coach holds the client as naturally creative, resourceful and whole. The agenda comes from the client and the coaching relationship addresses the client's whole life. Through a process of action and learning, the client makes desirable changes in one or more parts of his or her life to create a life that is fulfilling and balanced. On a practical level the coaching process addresses setting and achieving goals. On a spiritual level coaching leads to a purposeful life where actions flow from innermost values. The ultimate goal is supporting the client to reach her or his full potential.

Colon Health Care

Colon hydrotherapy is a safe and effective irrigation to remove toxic waste from the large intestine without the use of drugs. Filtered water and regulated temperatures soften and loosen waste, resulting in evacuation through natural peristalsis. Colonic can be helpful for such problems as constipation, psoriasis, acne, allergies, headaches and can improve overall health. Therapists may use abdominal massage during this process and advise the client regarding nutrition, fluids and exercise to enhance the colonic procedure and general health of the colon. Today's sophisticated technology promotes both safety and sanitation of the popular practice with the use of FDA equipment, disposable rectal nozzles and certified therapists.

Consegrity®

Consegrity is a self-healing approach for wellness. The balance and flow of energy fields in our body can determine our state of health, how we live and for how long. The Consegrity Wellness Model restores balance and supports all biological systems. Consegrity however is not a ticket to the spa, nor is it a quick fix for all your problems. The "facilitator" or "therapist" is your tour guide, helping you find the best route for your health. The journey can include stops at places in you that can be the source of energy and vitality. The Consegrity clinician guides the journey by holding a "map" or "mirror" to help the healing process. Consegrity is a very effective technique to open the door to what's possible in the human body's ability to heal.

Craniosacral Therapy

The craniosacral system surrounds the brain and the spinal cord. The practitioner utilizes the subtle rhythm of spinal fluid motion as it is transmitted along fascial planes throughout the body. Craniosacral therapy is a system of evaluation and light touch that views the individual as an integrated totality. Conditions that frequently respond well to this therapeutic modality include: acute musculo-skeletal injuries, chronic pain conditions associated with accidents and stress-exacerbated dysfunctions of the autonomic-nervous system.

Doula

A Doula is a woman experienced in childbirth who provides continuous physical, emotional and informational support to the mother before, during and just after childbirth. Trained Doulas understand the physiology of birth and the emotional needs of a woman in labor. Generally Doulas believe that pregnancy and birth are normal, natural and healthy processes. This includes preparation for birth, helping the laboring woman with encouragement, comfort measures, relaxation techniques and an objective viewpoint, as well as support after childbirth, such as help with breast-feeding.

Facial Rejuvenation

Facial Rejuvenation is a combination of massage and energy work. It assists nerve, muscle and energy reconnection through the use of select contact points and employs specific massage strokes and massage patterns to relax the muscles and increase circulation and energy flow to the face, neck, shoulders and head. This combined result allows a realignment of the facial muscles into a more stress-free, relaxed and youthful pattern. The treatment includes herbal compressing, cleansing, natural masks and may also utilize aromatherapy, with individually chosen aromatic essential oils, helping to move the body into a state of balance.

Falun Dafa

Falun Dafa, also known as Falun Gong, is a Chinese self-cultivation practice that improves mental and physical wellness though five easy-to-learn exercises, meditation and development of one's heart/ mind nature (Xinxing). The practice is based on the principles of Truthfulness-Compassion-Tolerance. This ancient form of Qigong, originally taught in private, was first introduced to the public in China in 1992, by Mr. Li Hongzhi. An important tenet of Falun Dafa is that all exercise instruction and activities are free of charge.

Feng Shui

Feng Shui (pronounced "fung shway") is the terrestrial equivalent of astrology and is the ancient mystical art of Chinese geomancy, studying the dynamic relationship between humans and the surrounding environment. It attempts to show how everybody can match their personal characteristics to their surroundings, whether at home or at work, thus ensuring greater environmental harmony and leading to enhanced inner peace.

Homeopathy

Homeopathy is derived from the Greek word homoio, meaning like or similar. This natural system of medicine was developed over 200 years ago by Samuel Hahneman, a German physician. It bases its practice on treating like with like. This homeopathic principle is based on treating an illness with a substance that produces, in a healthy person, similar symptoms to those experienced by the sick person, employing minute doses of natural remedies that are created from herbal, mineral and animal substances. Homeopathy views symptoms as the body's natural reaction in fighting the illness and, unlike conventional medicine, seeks to stimulate them rather than suppress them.

Hypnobirthing

Hypnobirthing classes teach self-hypnosis to expectant mothers and their partners. Couples learn proven, effective relaxation techniques to eliminate fear, tension and pain. Hypnobirthing parents achieve birth fulfillment, awake and alert, in a totally relaxed state of mind and body, often free of pain and without the need for medication. Birth and bonding are returned to the peaceful, serene manner of nature.

Hypnosis

Hypnotherapy is a technique that uses hypnosis to reach into the subconscious mind for solutions to problems with which the conscious mind has been unable to deal. The altered state occurring under hypnosis is akin to a state of deep meditation, where the recuperative abilities of the psyche are allowed to flow more freely. Hypnosis is a waking state, the hypnotized person remains in full control of his or her behavior and usually is able to recall the whole experience. Hypnotherapy has been used to treat addictions, relieve stress and help individuals develop a more positive attitude in general.

Imago Therapy

Imago relationship therapy recognizes that the inherent nature of human beings is what Carl G. Jung described as a "push toward wholeness." Throughout our development as human beings that wholeness is fragmented through experiences in relationship with our caretakers and results in significant impact on the choice of a marriage or relationship partner (the imago). Since unmet needs from childhood are brought into adult intimate partnerships for resolution, childhood frustrations are inevitably reactivated and experienced. These relational conflicts are an unconscious attempt by partners to finish childhood, reestablish contact without losing their identity and to recover a sense of wholeness.

Iridology

Iridology is the analysis of the iris of the eye, the colored portion that reveals the basic constitutional health of an individual.

Iridology can indicate genetic and functional weaknesses, tissue and organ condition, areas of nutritional depletion and need, areas of inflammation and toxicity and the general body constitution. This information is gathered by "reading" the fiber and markings of the iris, which manifests symptoms specific to all the organs of the body before they would be discernible through lab analysis or blood work.

Jin Shin Jyutsu

Jin Shin Jyutsu (Physio-Philosophy) is an ancient art of harmonizing the life energy in the body. Jin Shin Jyutsu employs 26 "safety energy locks" along energy pathways that feed life into our bodies. When one or more of the paths become blocked, the resulting stagnation can disrupt the local area and eventually dis-harmonize the complete path of energy flow. Holding these energy locks, by placing the fingertips (over clothing) on designated energy locks, restore the energy flow, bringing balance to mind, body and spirit.

Naturopathy

Naturopathy is a compilation of a wide variety of natural therapeutics and healing techniques. This natural method of healing is based on the premise that the body contains the innate wisdom and power to heal itself, providing that we enhance, rather than hinder, that process and in addition that treating the whole person is more desirable than simply alleviating the symptoms of disease. The Naturopathic physician utilizes such therapies as non-invasive allergy testing, herbology, acupressure, acupuncture and iridology.

Osteopathy

Osteopathy is a scientifically based philosophy of health care that embraces the concept of the interrelatedness of structure (anatomy) and function (physiology). Dysfunction of the musculo-skeletal system contributes to imbalances and insufficiencies of the circulation and nervous system, rendering the body vulnerable to disease. Osteopathic manual treatment of the musculo-skeletal system allows normal function to resume. Doctors of osteopathy are fully licensed physicians, who use the principles of osteopathy, along with traditional medical models, to promote the health of their patients.

Pilates

Pronounced "Puh-lah-tees," this "intelligent" exercise was developed by German nurse and fitness guru Joseph Pilates, after World War I, to assist bedridden patients in recovering muscle strength. The system employs specialized machines to teach the body self-awareness and strengthen muscles without straining them, in a complete and balanced way. Pilates has proven beneficial for the rehabilitation of injuries and is favored by dancers and athletes for muscle toning.

Polarity Therapy

One of the first Western therapy systems to utilize energy and understand that it is the bottom line of healing. Polarity was developed by Randolph Stone, osteopath, chiropractor and naturopath. It uses physical touch and pressure to balance energy in the body, conceiving of energy as flowing outward from a central core in the body, which is a reservoir of wholeness and health. Understanding the relationships between this energetic source within the body and the various flows of energy underlying physiological function, polarity helps the body restore itself to health based on its own resources. Polarity makes

97

use of these therapeutic sessions, as well as diet, self-awareness and energy based exercises.

Pranic Healing

Pranic healing is a form of bio-energy healing that focuses on accelerating the body's own ability to heal itself. By working on the bioplasmic body, we create a new pattern for the physical counterpart to follow, causing the body to heal much more rapidly. Pranic healing involves practical steps to remove energetic blockages and rapidly boost the life force of the affected parts.

Qigong

Qigong means "energy practice". These ancient chinese exercises generally consist of one or a few simple movements, done repetitively, focusing mind and breath through the body in specific ways. There are innumerable forms of Qigong, for general health and well-being, for healing specific organs or illnesses and for cultivating special capacities, from memory and extrasensory perceptions, to the highest spiritual development.

Reiki

In Reiki, a practitioner's hands are very gently placed on the fully-clothed body of a person in a variety of established places, on the head, chest, abdomen and back. This scientific method of activating and balancing the life-force energy (also known as prana, qi, or chi) was brought to the West in 1937 by Saici Takata. Light hand placement is used on the body in order to align the chakras and channel energy to organs and glands. Reiki can be used as a form of health maintenance and disease prevention, used as a self-help technique or on others.

Rolfing

Rolfing is a holistic system of connective tissue manipulation and movement education that systematically aligns, balances and integrates the whole body in gravity.

Sacred Geometry

Sacred geometry is the study of proportional root harmonies and the pattern language of nature's Sacred Principles of harmony, geometric shapes, music and art and how they are applied to human habitation and architectural form, to promote harmony by design.

Smart Bells

Smart bells are sculptural weights that blend Eastern and Western concepts of fitness. The weights are ergonomic, aerodynamic and aesthetic. Smart bells conform to the shape of the body and remain balanced in the circular movements of the routines. Smart bells break the "rules" of traditional weight lifting involving flow. Learn the 10 Core Exercises for functional fitness moving on to improvisation. In partner and group exercises, you "literally connect with others." Smart bells are fun, effective and inspire creativity.

Structural Integration

Structural Integration is a unique, whole systems approach to connective-tissue manipulation and movement education, created by the late biochemist and physiologist Dr. Ida P. Rolf. The work is defined by the intelligent process and guiding principles of rebalancing the human body in relation to itself and gravity. Structural integration blends science (anatomy) with art (hands-on manipulation), allowing the practitioner to skillfully unwind the postural compensations and distortions that so often lead to chronic pain and physiological dysfunction.

Tai Chi Chu'an/Qi Gong

The forms of Tai Chi Chuan are a traditional chinese approach to exercise, meditation and personal growth. Practiced both for health and self-defense, it's graceful, flowing movements are beautiful, healthful and powerful. It's practice promotes an inner calm and a tranquil attitude, enhancing self-awareness.

Tai Chi springs from emptiness and is born of nature. It is the source of motion and tranquility and the mother of Yin and Yang. The body weight, or center of gravity of the practitioner, sinks into the abdomen and trunk of the body, thus allowing more relaxed and deep breathing. With the mind quieted, the heartbeat slows down and different muscular, neurological, glandular and organ systems function in a more balanced fashion. The practice of Tai Chi Chuan is harmony and understanding of the ways of the world.

Thermography

Breast thermography is a painless, noninvasive clinical test that gives women the opportunity to increase their chances of detecting breast disease at an early stage. With this test there is no contact with the body and no exposure to radiation. A breast tumor has often been growing 8 to 10 years before it is dense enough to show up on a mammogram. Thermography picks up physiological changes that are present in early stages of tumor growth, thereby giving women the opportunity to intervene years earlier to reverse changes and regain breast health.

Yoga

Yoga is an ancient Indian practice that is a scientific system designed to bring the practitioners' health, happiness and a greater sense of Self. In Yoga the body and mind are linked to create a state of internal peacefulness and integration. At the practical level and included in the contemporary definitions of Yoga, are the actual physiological/mental techniques themselves. These techniques concentrate on posture and alignment, as well as creating a higher consciousness. Yoga utilizes stretching postures, breathing and meditation techniques to calm the emotional state and the mind and tone the body to a greater sense of Self. At the practical level and included in the contemporary definitions of Yoga, are the actual physiological/mental techniques themselves. These techniques concentrate on posture and alignment, as well as creating a higher consciousness.

WHAT YOUR FEET CAN TELL YOU ABOUT YOUR HEALTH

A natural healthy body has beautifully formed feet, free of callouses and blemishes. Balanced in their view of their inherent tendency, is to be flexible so that they can confidently stride ahead with love and joy, adapting spontaneously and appropriately to every situation. Feet sympathetically tune into thoughts and respond accordingly. The marks of life's experiences impress the soul and the sole and are reflected on feet long before being mirrored in the physical body. Distortions of the feet outwardly display distortions and misconceptions of the mind. Disharmony from mental confusion and emotional turmoil is projected into the physical body, causing disease, pain and anxiety, reflecting an unhappy state of mind. Thoughts of fear, hate and envy create tension, havoc and confusion, while loving thoughts relax the mind, body and soul, harmonising all bodily systems. It is easier to replace uneasy thought patterns with healthy ones and Reflexology provides the option to choose again to create that different experience. A change of mind lifts individuals from limiting circumstances and places them on a journey of self-discovery, with a life that contains all the elements of happiness.

As the foot represents all parts of the body, it is important to treat the feet with care, washing regularly and do remember to be careful about drying between the toes to prevent cracks developing. Always use a pumice stone and some cream to help soften hardened areas, such as corns, verrucas and athlete's foot. The person to deal with these problems is a chiropodist.

Feet should be kept warm and comfortable at all times and give a little pamper from time to time. Treat the feet well and they will look after you.

BEING POSITIVE ABOUT YOUR THINKING

When we are positive all around us will be positive. It is amazing what happens when we are in this frame of mind: what we give out we get back. Likewise when we are negative this will spread to others because we are creating a negative atmosphere. Nobody needs a negative person. It has been proven that when we are positive people enjoy having us in their company. When we are in a positive frame of mind we feel good in ourselves and our health improves. When we are in bad form, moaning and feeling doom and gloom, this is all we get back from others. When we are at dis-ease, we have disease. Always remember: it only takes one smile to make thousands of others smile.

FEMALE & MALE MENOPAUSE

Menopause means the time when menstruation stops. The age of menopause can average from as early as 30's to late 50's. This is a time when many problems can occur. Thankfully today more and more women are getting medical advice for their menstrual and menopause symptoms, in the past women did not know what was going on in their own body and system. During menopause women would have night "sweats", which are very distressing, they feel anxious, tense and some get panic attacks, mood swings and palpitations. This is caused by changes in the hormones or chemical substances secreted in the body. Hormones play such a huge part in a woman's life and when these changes occur, men do not realise how difficult it can be to accept the changes in her body, men often think the woman is simply going crazy.

Men and women are so different, for example, when a woman is upset she wants and needs to talk, but the man just wants to read the newspaper or go for a pint, leading to bad feeling and resentment for both. Women should know that these symptoms will eventually pass, but would will be able to deal with them easier with a little understanding, help and some relaxing therapy.

Also men go through menopause. One sign noticed when some men are going through is the desire to go hunting again, looking for a younger woman to make them feel good or wanting to buy a sport car, changing their hair style, etc. A man then begins to complain about his wife, saying she does not do this or that and there is nothing left between them. He will accuse her of always arguing, not listening to him, that she does not understand him. He will say their relationship has long gone and they no longer communicate. He blames her for nagging and looks for a new woman who will understand and feel sorry for him. All those things he finds fault with in his wife are seldom true. He thinks his wife does not see what is happening, while really women have extremely good intuition. A wife will know by her husbands' actions what is going on, most wives will try to tolerate what is happening and be supportive, in the hope that he will get through this stage of his life and will realise what he has. Thankfully not all men going through male menopause feel the need to go hunting and instead a man realises what he has and works through this time of his life with the support of his wife and family. What a wonderful world it would be if only women and men could understand each other a little better.

RESPONSIBILITY FOR OUR OWN HEALTH

Long ago people had to find their own cures for illness, particularly people with families who possibly had no work and would not be in a position to pay for doctors and medication, as money was more scarce. Years ago most people grew their own vegetables and potatoes, there was so much less pollution, drinking water was cleaner, hospital super bugs were unheard of, people were less stressed than today. But it's time now to take our own health into our own hands. One way to do that is through our feet. Our feet connect us to the ground, but they also represent our connection between our earthly and spiritual life, they ground us literally and figuratively. They are our base and foundation and our contact with the earth and the energies that flow through it. They can also play a major role in attaining and maintaining better health and well-being. Healing begins when we start to love ourselves. We need to be in tune with the physical, spiritual and emotional. We have to have control over the quality of our life. This is the body I happen to be in, so I have to take care of it by leaving it open to healing itself. It is important for you to let go of tension and to trust your own ability to visualise the healing power within you. Accept yourself as you are and try to do a little relaxation each day. We all need a little stress in our lives, but remember there are two types of stress, the good and the bad. We need to get rid of the bad by controlling it, this is not always easy, but it has to go. We do not value our health until it's gone. Our health is our wealth. Our bodies are mirrored in our feet, so let us look after our feet, they are our warning signs.

OLD CURES FROM THE PAST

Our mothers learned and believed in the "old cures" passed on from their own mothers and grandmothers. The belief was that every plant that grew around them had the property to cure:

Nettles: were used to make a nourishing soup with a mixture of whatever vegetable were available, expecially in mid / late summer, when nettles grow abudantly in places where the electromagnetic field is strong. The nettles can give you a sting, however the sting is good for arthritic hands and arthritis of the joints.

Thyme: which blooms between early and late summer, can be used both in cooking and in the treatment of illnesses. A cup of thyme tea in the morning, instead of regular tea, can work wonders for your stomach.

Rice: fill a clean sock with a cup of uncooked rice, tie off the top of the sock and heat it up, wrap this warm sock around any painful joint and it will make the pain go away.

Sea salt: another help for joint pain is to add sea salt to a warm bath and relax in the water.
For sore throat: years ago they used to get a silk stocking, put salt into the stocking and heat it up, then it would be wrapped gently around the neck at bedtime and, sure enough, next morning the throat would be much better.
For sweaty feet: use warm water with salt in it and soak the feet, the salt helps harden the pores in the feet.

Sugar and Red Soap: put some red soap and sugar on a piece of lint and put on a sore heel or stone bruise. Years ago children had to go bare-footed and were prone to stone bruising and sore feet.

Tea Bags: allows two used tea bags to cool, then close your eyes, put the tea bags on them for ten minutes. This is good for tired eyes.

Potato: men were known to carry a potato, or a copper coin in their pocket, to relieve the pain of arthritis.

Lemon Juice: use a squeeze of lemon juice for 2-3 days on a corn and it will peel away.

Bread: this was used as a "poultice" which would draw boils or whittles. The poultice was made by placing a small piece of white bread onto a piece of gauze and pouring boiling water over the bread. The gauze was then wrapped around the boil or whittle until it burst.

Vinegar: put vinegar straight onto a sting and the pain goes away.

FIFTH SECTION

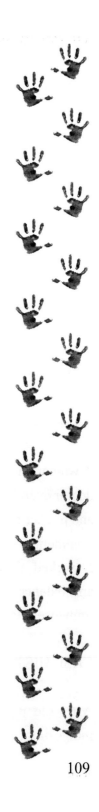

CASE HISTORY

Since becoming a reflexologist, I have seen so many amazing things happen when people come for treatments. Through the years I have seen so many people walk through the door with long faces, feeling depressed, sore, angry, in pain and simply not knowing what was wrong with them. I have seen these same people after a few, or even sometimes just one treatment, walk out the door with head held high, feeling better in themselves and about themselves. I have seen them leave looking and feeling peaceful, in harmony and with a better attitude to life.

These cases that follow are some exemples of my time as reflexologist:

CASE HISTORY 1 - DIZZINESS

A woman in her late 30's was suffering from a lot of dizziness. Her doctor examined her ears and told her she was suffering from vertigo and put her on medication, which did help. She came for reflexology treatment to see if it could improve her condition.

I worked the area to the pituitary, neck, head, eustacion tube and balance points. The woman felt her state of health improved immensely through the benefit of reflexology.

CASE HISTORY 2 - INDIGESTION

A 67 old man, with a very responsible job, suffered a lot with indigestion, especially after rich meals, which he constantly had

110

when out on business lunches. His mother had told him about reflexology and he decided to have a few treatments, which he thoroughly enjoyed and his problem improved. I also taught him how to work on his hand when he got indigestion, so he could work on the stomach and oesophagus reflexes to give himself relief.

CASE STUDY 3 - ASTHMA

An extremely rewarding case was one of a little girl, aged 7, who had suffered with severe asthma. Her mother asked whether reflexology would give her child any relief, as her quality of life was extremely impaired. The child was treated on a regular basis and there were gradual improvements by the end of one month.

CASE STUDY 4 - BACKACHE

A 50 year old lady complained with stiffening in her back. Working down the spine, I found the lower lumbar area extremely tender, also the side of the neck, which was picked up touching the side of the big toes was tender. Having worked on both feet for about an hour, paying special attention to the spine and neck, the lady felt much relief and looking forward to her next treatment.

CASE STUDY 5 - PAINFUL PERIODS

A 15 year old girl was having very painful periods and after treatment for the reproductive organs, she had great relief thereafter. One has to go very lightly on the reproductive organs, also keep in mind that children need a shorter treatment.

CASE STUDY 6 - PREGNANCY

C.G. came to me for a reflexology section. While she was relaxing, with her eyes closed during the treatment, I placed my hands on her stomach. C.G. felt immense heat and was amazed to clearly picture an image of her uterus with her baby inside. She stated: "This was an extremely beautiful and moving experience"; she did not realise she was pregnant until I told her. A month later she returned and confirmed to me that she was indeed pregnant.

One of the amazing things of doing reflexology on a mother who is pregnant is that the baby feels when the therapist puts her hands on the mother's feet. The baby feels a bit uneasy at first but after a while it settles down and is very quiet; but when the hands are taken off the mother's feet the baby gets disturbed again, so it's better to take off the hands gradually.

CASE STUDY 7 - INFFERTILITY

L.A. married for many years, but infertile, was "desperate" when she came for reflexology. She found the first session soothing and relaxing and felt "very positive" after it. She had continuing regular treatments and particular attention was paid to the reproductive system, which left her with feelings of physical and emotional strength. She was thrilled to discover she was pregnant after so long and continued treatments throughout the pregnancy. She gave birth of a healthy baby boy who loves holding his parents feet. This usually happens when the mother receives reflexology treatments while pregnant. Not only was it helping her but also the baby.

CASE STUDY 8 - LYMPH DRAINAGE

M. was in her 70s when she had a bad fall, splitting her head open and causing enormous damage to her leg, which then became severely infected. With her knowledge of reflexology, M. was able to help herself with particular reference to the lymph drainage. She had to attend hospital for daily dressings and the medical staff there were amazed at her rapid recovery, particularly considering her age. M. gives full credit to reflexology for this. It was great that she knew what to do for herself. No harm having a bit of knowledge about Reflexology.

CASE STUDY 9 - ANXIETY

A young man came for reflexology treatment as he was suffering from anxiety. He was very nervous and restless and could not settle down to study. I explained what I was doing and he was happy to leave things in my hands, as he felt he could trust me.
He told me he was a twin and always had the feeling that his other twin was pushing him out, which had affected him since his childhood. After a course of treatments his life got good for him and he has never looked back.

CASE STUDY 10 - BACK PAIN

A man in his 50s had a problem with the lower back area and when the pain became excruciating, he finally decided to try reflexology. I found sensitivity in the left kidney area and both the right and left urethra tubes, due to retention of urine. During treatment the man

113

was so relaxed and fell asleep. When he woke up he was amazed at how good he felt. The next day he call me to say he had passed so much urine and he felt so much improved.

CASE STUDY 11 - KIDNEY INFECTION

A young lady had a history of kidney infections, which had troubled her for many years. Every so often, she would experience excruciating pain and would visit her doctor, who would put her on medication, which would help for a few weeks. The morning after the reflexology treatment she phoned to say she was feeling so much better and would continue with the sections. Her kidneys were very tender to touch and after each session she would pass a lot of water, which was darker and stronger. This lady was on medication every time she got an infection in her kidneys. Since she has got reflexology she has not had any trouble for the last 2 years. She continues with the reflexology treatments. She is also a more relaxed person, so her husband and children tell her.

CASE STUDY 12 - CANCER

A lady, 38 years old, had very bad health. All her life she smoked about 30 cigarettes a day. She tried to kick the habit but to no avail. A year ago she was diagnosed with having lung cancer. She decided not to have medical treatment, but to proceed with the natural route. She is very positive and gives no room to the negative, she eats all fresh vegetables and fruit. Now she is having Reflexology, she finds it very calming and it helps her to sleep better than she has been. Each morning she says "I will kill the cancer before it kills me". She tries to live a stress free life as much as she can. She firmly believes in Reflexology and gets a source of energy from it. This lady has great faith and believes "there is a time to live and a time to die".

She wonders why doctors don't use Reflexology alongside conventional medicine. Hopefully it will come some day when they will work in tandem for the good of all.

CASE STUDY 13 - SINUSITIS and BACKACHE

A lady with some health problems came to me. She did not smoke, would take alcohol only occasionally, she was a vegetarian and conscious of her diet. She was suffering frequently from sinusitis and backache. She would feel tired in the evenings but sleeping well at night. This lady previously had Reflexology from a friend, but she decided to have another try from someone else, so she came to me and, on examining her feet, I noticed a lot of hard skin on the shoulder area. As I worked on this area I felt there was discomfort in both feet and very tender in the chest area.

She suffered from regular colds and was currently on medication for her chest. She was quite open to any influence that Reflexology may have. When I worked on her feet she fell asleep for about 30 minutes. She spoke about the energy she felt as I was working on her, she found that my hands were so warm, she said it was like a heater. I explained that sometimes energy gets blocked in the body and that Reflexology breaks down these blockages in the system, which prevents the body from working properly.

CASE STUDY 14 - DEPRESSION

I met a friend of mine who was telling me about her son who was suffering from depression. The signs and symptoms of depression are many and varied and may rob one of energy and ability to make decisions. My friend did not know what to do with him, so

I asked if he had gotten treatment for his depression, she told me he had but was no better. She asked me to have a talk with him, as she would like him to try to have Reflexology done. I told her I would do my best for him but that he must first mention to his doctor and to get the go ahead from him, which he did.

After a few treatments of Reflexology the young man made a recovery, was sleeping much better and had a bad day only now and again. When this would happen he phoned me and I gave him time to talk and gave him a treatment of Reflexology. He called it his little fix and found it relaxing, which he needed.

Listening, and I mean really listening to what is going on in the person's mind and then treating the real cause is what heals.

CASE STUDY 15 - EMPHYSEMA

A client who was attending Reflexology for migraine, spoke to me about her mother who was extremely ill with emphysema, which as we know, causes the lungs to lose their elasticity, due to the alveolar walls collapsing, greatly reducing the surface area for gaseous interchange to take place. She explained that her mother had difficulty breathing out, leaving air trapped in the diseased airways and causing her to become distressed. When this happens

116

the chest is elevated by the accessory muscles of respiration and the diaphragm becomes flattened. Unfortunately there is not a lot can be done, apart from medically trying to control the symptoms with steroids, to break down the excessive inflammation in the lungs and anti-diuretic tablets, to try to control the fluid in the lung area. I explained that this medication can cause side effects and perhaps a little reflexology relaxation would help. When my client brought her mother to me, I worked on her feet with 2 fingers down the nervous system, working with my 2 thumbs back and forward across the chest and lung area with light strokes. The lady became very relaxed and found it much easier to breathe.

CASE STUDY 16 - HYPOTHYROIDISM

Hypothyrodism, or low thyroid function, is one of the most widely suffered and least detected illness, a silent saboteur of health and morale. I did reflexology treatments on a lady who had a very notable thyroid. After working on her feet for about 5 weeks, I could see the lump on the neck being reduced. Her doctor was considering an operation, but after the reflexology treatments, the doctor was very pleased with her progress. This lady had a very busy lifestyle, with a very important job and just did not have the time to look after herself, so she stopped coming for Reflexology, although she believed in it. As she could not have it both ways, her thyroid increased in size after she ceased the treatments. No doubt this lady will come again when it is too late, looking for a miracle. Reflexology does work, but you have to given it time.

CASE STUDY 17 - TERMINALLY ILL

One woman, who had a brain tumor, was recommended Reflexology as a way to relax. When I went to see her, she was extremelly agitated and naturally didn't want to die. Over the 10 months of her illness, I got to know my client very well and she looked forward to our little time together. Touching her feet I could feel they were clammy and stiff, discoloured in parts, particularly around the big toe. I could feel her tension through my hands, but, by touching her feet, I got her to relax so that during most of the treatment my client would fall asleep and her whole face would loose it's furrows of pain. After the treatment I was so pleased to see the contentment in her face and sense of well-being. She was pleased to know that I was someone who really cared for her confort. Many clients I treated felt they could cope better with their chemoteraphy and radiation following a session of Reflexology, as it calms the system and lessen the tiredness and anxiety.

CASE STUDY 18 - SHINGLES (Herpes Zoster)

The virus that causes chicken pox in children seems responsible for shingles, an infection of a major spinal nerve, which semicircles the body and brings with it severe neuralgic pain and skin rash. Adults exposed to children with chicken pox often become infected with shingles and vice versa. Apparently adults who have had chicken pox carry the dormant virus, which can fare into action when the immune system defences are weak.

I did reflexology on a few people, after being medically treated and after the shingles settled down. Their health improved quicker, due to the effect of Reflexology in boosting the immune system.

CASE HISTORY 19 - TINNITUS

This problem has been described as hearing a constant, annoying tortouring noise, day and night. J. came to Reflexology after a suggestion from his wife and after four treatments he was amazed at the impruvement that occured in that very short time.

CASE STUDY 20 - DUODOENAL ULCER - letter

In December 1996 I was diagnosed with having a duodenal ulcer and my doctor recommended that I attend for Reflexology with Sr. Brega to help me "de-stress". At that time I had no idea what Reflexology was and in fact, if I had been told that it involved working with my feet, I would not have attended, I, as with a lot of people I know, felt that someone touching my feet would only make me start giggling. Sr. Brega told me to lie down on the reflexology couch, placed a support cushion under my knees and started to work on my feet. Instead of feeling any tickling sensation, all I felt was gentle pressure on all areas of my feet. Within seconds Sr. Brega told me that I was having problems with my stomach area, which surprised me since I had not told her why I was attending for Reflexology. During the course of my treatment Sr. Brega also told me several things which were "out of order" in my body, i.e. back complaint, sinus trouble and an ovarian problem, all of which were proven true over the next few years. When my treatment was finished, I was so relaxed and lethargic that all I wanted to do was stay where I was. By the time I got home, all the dreadful sensation of choking I had from the ulcer had disappeared.

Over the years I have attended Sr. Brega any time I feel in any way "under the weather" and have always walked out on air. Not only has Reflexology helped me where medical problems have arisen, but has helped me to be a more relaxed and patient person.

I have recommended Reflexology to so many of my friends and colleagues and never once has it failed. Thank you Sr. Brega.

Bernadette

CASE STUDY 21 - LUPUS - letter

In the summer of 1992 I was living and working in Boston, when I suddenly became ill with very severe pain in my major joints.

I was diagnosed with S.L.E (more commonly known as Lupus).

I was referred to a rheumatologist in Massachusetts general hospital who, after examing me, wanted to prescribe medications to slow down the disease. Howewer there were many side effects, one of which was possible infertility. I was wery upset by this as I had always wanted children. The doctor's words were that I would most likely be in a wheelchair within 6 months if I did not take the medication. I refused to start on this medication and moved back to Ireland, to live with my parents, I was unable to stay in the USA, as I could not work and had no medical insurance.

It was a very difficult time as myself and my family all tried to live with my illness. I was very depressed and angry as my condition continued to worsen. My hands had become curled and I was waiting for an operation to see if they could be straightened. I was attending for physiotherapy 3 times a week, but the tendons in my hands had become like marbles, so the physio was no longer working. I had to wear casts on my hands at night and bandages by day to try to stop them from getting any worse. During this bad time I had my first experience of body and spirit: my spirit so badly wanted the old me back, but the body just was not able. I prayed so hard for the pain to go away, but nothing happened.

In summer 1994 my prayers were answered by a chance meeting: my mother sat beside a lady on a bus and they started to talk. The lady told my mom she was about to visit her niece in hospital, who was suffering from a disese called Lupus. The lady told her about Sr. Brega and Reflexology and gave my mum Sr. Brega's number. That chance meeting was about to change my life. At this stage of my illness my mother had to help me wash and dress.

On my first visit to Sr. Brega, she explained Reflexology to me as she worked. It took all my strenght to climb up on the bed and I was in a lot of pain, as she worked for a couples of hours, but it felt like a "good pain". I slept for hours after my first tratment and returned the following day for Sr. Brega to work again as I fell in and out of sleep. At one stage she was working on my hands, when she asked me to open my eyes. Next thing I knew my hands were opening like flowers in bloom and I could not believe my eyes, my hands were perfectly straight for the first time over a year. Sr. Brega continued to work on me for the next few months, until all my symptons were gone. I take no medication and it has now been 12 years sice I was first diagnosed. I have had a few relapses since then, but I went for few treatments to get me back on track. I have never looked back since my first experience with Reflexology and Sr. Brega and I am delighted to say I am now married to George and the mother of a beautiful 3 year old daugther called Kayleigh. I know in my heart that the meeting on the no. 31 bus, all those years ago, was no chance, it was fate and an the answer to my prayer.

Maureen

CONCLUSION

My theory is that once you get a body to relax it will heal itself. If you feel a person is too ill to give a full treatment to, they can benefit from a little light relaxation all over the feet, always worthwhile, but ensure the client tells their doctor about having Reflexology. Most doctors will say, get whatever will help you.

Reflexology provides a different experience that involves a change of mind that lifts individuals from limiting circumstances and places them on a journey of self-discovery, with a life that contains all the elements of happiness.

Mothers in particular feel "guilty" giving themselves a little treat, but I have seen so many mothers feel like the weight of the world has been lifted off their shoulders after Reflexology. A little relaxation is very good for all of us, so whatever therapy makes you happy go for it! Lighten up. Laugh more. Make time for yourself, your family and friends. Most of all live life and don't let it pass you by.

For informations about Registerd Reflexologists in Ireland visit:
www.nationalreflexology.ie

or e-mail:
info@nationalreflexology.ie

ACKNOWLEDGEMENTS

A heartfelt thank you to all who helped and supported me in creating this book. Thanks for their encouragement, effort, hard work and their belief in me. In particular I would like to thank my valuable friends: Marian Barry, for the help when I first came up with the idea many years ago, Bernadette Keegan and Audrey Markey for their time and generosity. Many thanks and good wishes go to Jane Vukvic, course director of the Churchill College in London, with whom I had the pleasure of training in the 1980s. Also thanks to James for his help in the past and Liam for his encouragement. Thanks to Claudia for helping me in getting this book printed, for providing the illustrations and thanks also for your trust and belief in me.

I hope that all who read this book will benefit for it.
I wish you all good health and happiness.

Sr. Brega

ABOUT THE AUTHOR

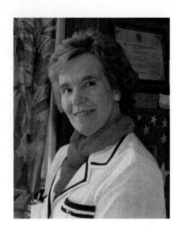

Sr. Brega Whelan is founder of the Beaumont Institute of Complementary Therepies. She has trained in many therapies like Biotherapy, Craneo Sacro Therepy, Kinesiology, etc. But her first love was, and still is Reflexology which she still teaches in Ireland.

Sr. Brega has had articles published in the journal for The National Register of Reflexologist and in newspapers in Ireland. She has been intervew in several radio and television programs.

Lightning Source UK Ltd.
Milton Keynes UK
178436UK00001B/166/P